P. J. Slootweg

Dental Pathology

Pieter J. Slootweg

Dental Pathology

A Practical Introduction

With 197 Figures

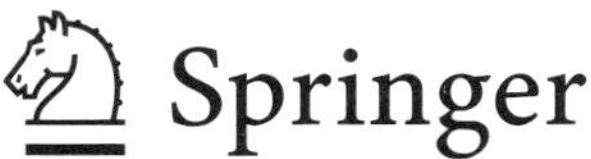

Pieter J. Slootweg, MD, DMD, PhD
Radboud University Medical Center Nijmegen
Department of Pathology
Huispost 824, 6500 HB
Nijmegen, Netherlands

Library of Congress Control Number: 2007923413

ISBN 978-3-540-71690-7 Springer Berlin Heidelberg New York

Springer is a part of Springer Science+Business Media

springer.com

Editor: Gabriele Schröder, Heidelberg, Germany
Desk Editor: Ellen Blasig, Heidelberg, Germany
Reproduction, typesetting and production: LE-TEX Jelonek, Schmidt & Vöckler GbR, Leipzig, Germany
Cover design: Frido Steinen-Broo, EStudio, Calamar, Spain

Printed on acid-free paper 24/3180/YL 5 4 3 2 1 0

Foreword

The textbook and atlas "Dental Pathology—A Practical Introduction" occupies a unique niche in dental-medical publishing. In fact, the book aims to be a substitute for the famous book "Pathology of dental hard tissues", written and edited by the late Jens J. Pindborg, Copenhagen, for which there has not been a successor for almost 40 years. Dental pathology primarily focussing on macro- and microstructure of teeth and adjacent tissues is very specific and fully understood only by those who specialise in this field or who have developed interest in the "Organon dentale". The author, Prof. Pieter J. Slootweg, Nijmegen, The Netherlands, has extensively been dealing with dental, oral, and maxillofacial pathology during his entire career. His expertise and lifelong experience with this specialty in pathology has resulted in an authoritative and encyclopaedic work presented in this book. The author has elegantly described what some consider a process difficult to understand, namely tooth formation. An overview about macro- and micro-disturbances of tooth form and dental hard structure is given. Also, the book deals with alterations acquired after tooth eruption, disturbed tooth eruption, disorders of dental pulp and periodontal tissues. In addition, the book extensively deals with odontogenic cysts and tumors.

Besides the concise text, an especially strong feature of the book is the many photomicrographs and clinical photos, which provide the reader with an unusual level of high quality visual documentation.

I truly believe that this book represents the most extensive review in the field and that it fills a gap in the dental and medical literature. It certainly should become a standard of reference for dental students as well as researchers in the field.

Berlin, March 2007
Prof. Dr. Peter A. Reichart

Preface

Diagnosis and treatment of diseases in the oral cavity is quite often hampered by the fact that this part of the human body is a subject of attention for two different branches of health care: medicine and dentistry. Therefore, there may be an overlap of both expertises in some areas but also neglect of others. An example of an area underdeveloped in the treatment of patients with diseases of the oral cavity is the adequate diagnostic application of knowledge of the gross and microscopical appearances exhibited by afflictions of the teeth and their surrounding structures. Pathologists with their medical training are in general not familiar with the basic anatomy and histology of these tissues and thus lack the background knowledge required for proper assessment of the pathologic alterations that may occur therein. Oral surgeons and dentists of course have a vast experience in diagnosis and treatment of dental and related diseases but they in general do not have the laboratory facilities at their disposal needed for histopathology, nor the microscopical skill of the experienced pathologist.

This book intends to fill this gap by providing practically applicable knowledge on macroscopical and histological changes that are seen in diseases of the dental and periodontal tissues. The aim is to enable the pathologist to recognize and interpret alterations in teeth and periodontal tissues in such a way that the results from this investigation are useful for the clinician who has submitted the material. Moreover, the content of this book should enable the clinician to formulate specific questions on histological features that may be present to provide the pathologist with a guideline how to interpret the slides prepared from the tissue samples under investigation. In this way, the communication between clinician and pathologist will be facilitated, thus improving patient care.

As histopathology of teeth and adjacent tissues requires knowledge of the normal development and histology of the dentition, the book starts with two chapters devoted to these subjects. Thereafter, chapters discuss the gross and microscopical features of diseases of the teeth, either developmental or acquired. Then, chapters are devoted to disease of the periodontal tissues, odontogenic cysts, and odontogenic tumours. The final chapter discusses how to distinguish between odontogenic tumours and developing odontogenic tissues, an area fraught with difficulties and with severe consequences for the patient if this distinction is not drawn appropriately. As far as possible, descriptions and illustrations include gross features, as well as radiological and histological aspects. Where appropriate, also the appearances shown in ground sections are mentioned.

Nijmegen, the Netherlands, March 2007
Pieter J. Slootweg

Contents

Chapter 1

Tooth Formation

1

Teeth develop from epithelial cells from the mucosal lining of the oral cavity and cranial neural crest-derived ectomesenchymal cells. These latter cells originate at the ectodermal/neuroectodermal junction of the developing brain, extending rostrally from the caudal boundary of the hindbrain and neural tube to the midbrain and caudal forebrain. They give rise to most connective tissues in the craniofacial region including the bones of the calvarium, face, and jaws. Since these bones that are formed by mesenchymal cells have an ectodermal/neuroectodermal ancestry, they are also known as ectomesenchyme [4–7].

The process of tooth formation starts with the formation of the dental lamina, a sheet of epithelial cells extending from the lining of the oral cavity into the underlying ectomesenchyme. In this dental lamina, focal bud-like thickenings determine the sites of the future teeth, 20 for the deciduous dentition and 32 for the permanent one, and together with a surrounding aggregation of ectomesenchymal cells they represent the earliest stage of the tooth germ (Figs. 1.1a, 1.2).

Subsequently, the epithelial bud transforms into a cap and from that point on is called enamel organ. Due to the formation of a concavity along the inner surface, the cap transforms into a bell. Ectomesenchymal cells lying within this concavity form the dental papilla that will become the dental pulp, the soft tissue core of the teeth. Other ectomesenchymal cells surround the enamel organ and form the dental follicle, the fibrous bag that invests the tooth germ and separates it from the adjacent jaw bone. Within the bell-shaped enamel organ, three different components are discerned: the inner enamel epithelium facing the dental papilla, the outer enamel epithelium lying adjacent to the dental follicle, and the intervening loose stellate epithelium that is called the stellate reticulum (Figs. 1.1b, 1.3).

From the bell stage onwards, reciprocal inductive events take place causing inner enamel epithelium and adjacent dental papilla cells to develop into enamel-forming ameloblasts and dentin-producing odontoblasts. The differentiation of dental papilla cells into odontoblasts

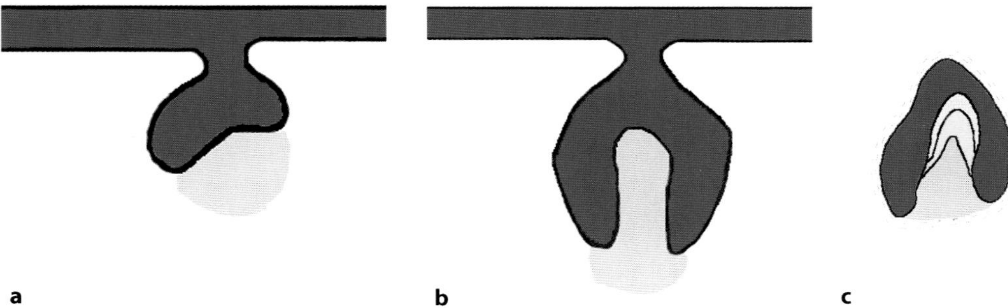

Fig. 1.1a–c Diagram showing consecutive stages of early tooth formation. **a** Bud stage, **b** Cap stage, and **c** Bell stage. Epithelium shown in *blue*, ectomesenchyme in *pink*, dentin in *yellow*, and enamel in *grey*

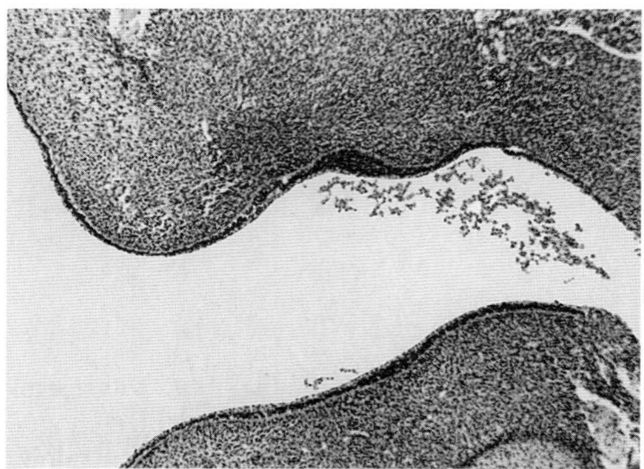

Fig. 1.2 Epithelial thickening of oral epithelium with underlying ectomesenchyme

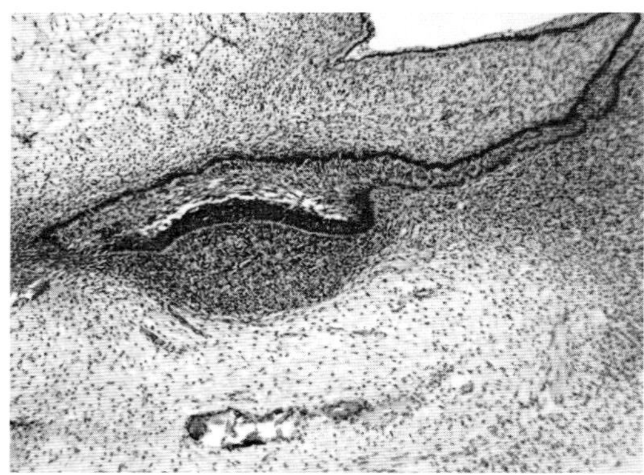

Fig. 1.3 Cap stage of tooth germ showing enamel organ composed of loose stellate reticulum bordered by inner enamel epithelium facing the ectomesenchymal condensation that will develop into the dental papilla (see Fig. 1.4)

requires a stimulus from the inner enamel epithelium, whereas the terminal differentiation of inner enamel epithelium into enamel-producing ameloblasts cannot occur without the presence of dentin. Therefore, dentin production occurs before enamel production and this is recapitulated in some odontogenic lesions that may display dentin formation but no enamel production, whereas the converse is never seen.

The odontoblasts form a matrix of collagen fibres called predentin that subsequently calcifies to become dentin. During dentinogenesis, odontoblasts recede from the dentino-enamel junction leaving a cytoplasmic extension behind in the deposited dentinal matrix. This explains why dentin has a tubular architecture, each dentinal tubule containing the cytoplasmic process of a single odontoblast (Figs. 1.1c, 1.4a, b).

Deposition of enamel starts after a tiny amount of dentin has been formed at the interface between future ameloblasts and odontoblasts. The enamel matrix subsequently calcifies to consist of approximately 95% minerals. This high mineral content explains why it does not withstand decalcification needed for histology.

While ameloblasts and odontoblasts are depositing enamel and dentin, inner and outer enamel epithelial cells join and proliferate in a downward way to encircle an increasing part of the dental papilla, thus creating a tube that maps out the form and size of the root of the teeth. This epithelial cuff is known as the epithelial root sheath or root sheath of Hertwig. In this root sheath, the inner enamel epithelium does not differentiate into enamel producing ameloblasts anymore but still induces the dental papilla cells to become odontoblasts that have to form the root dentin (Figs. 1.5, 1.6). Thereafter, Hertwig's root sheath fragmentates. In this way, ectomesenchymal cells from the dental follicle gain access to the root surface. These cells differentiate into cementoblasts and secrete cementoid on the surface of the intermediate cementum laid down before by them as an initial layer. Cementoid calcifies to become cementum. Whether cells from Hertwig's root sheath also contribute to initial cementum formation is controversial [1, 3, 8].

Besides the formation of cementum, dental follicle ectomesenchymal cells are also responsible for the formation of the other periodontal tissues: parts of the bony alveolar socket and the collagenous periodontal ligament that connects the tooth with this socket.

Remnants of Hertwig's root sheath form a permanent component of the periodontal ligament; they are known as rests of Malassez and are the source of some cystic jaw lesions. Moreover, these epithelial rests probably play a role in preventing contact between root surface and alveolar socket bone, thus ensuring preservation of tooth mobil-

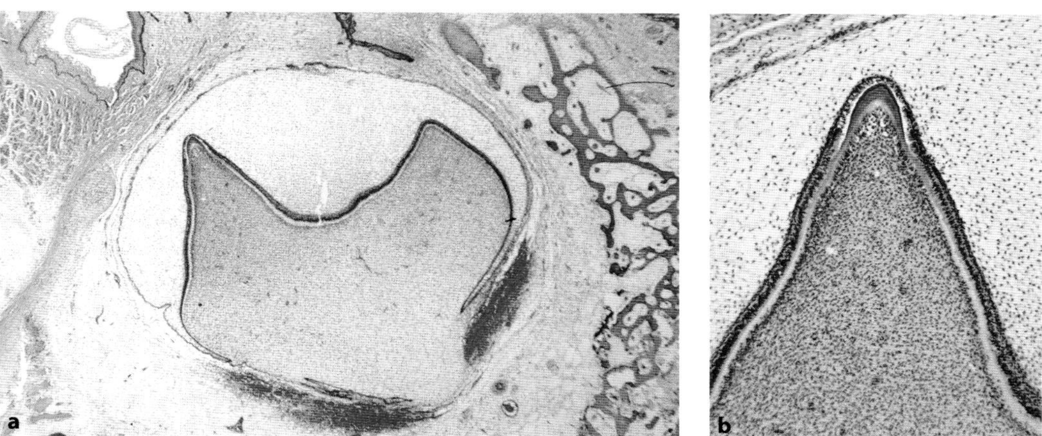

Fig. 1.4 **a** Bell stage of tooth germ. **b** At the tip of the dental papilla, deposition of enamel (*purple*) and dentin (*pink*) has started

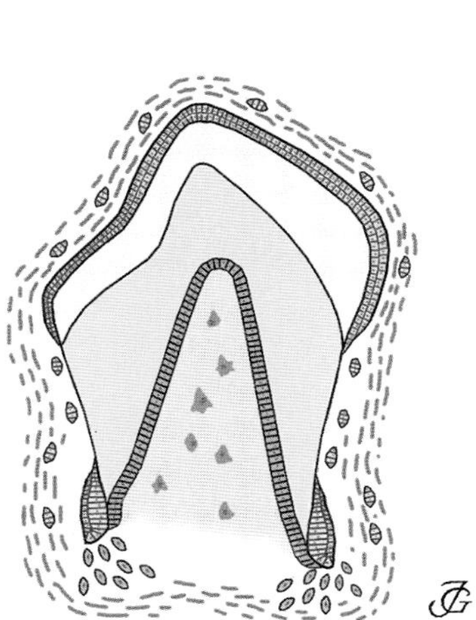

Fig. 1.5 Tooth germ in its late development. The crown is completely formed. The root is still growing at its apical tip, cells from the dental papilla being recruited to become dentin-forming odontoblasts. At this site, inner enamel epithelium still induces development of odontoblasts with subsequent dentin formation, but the subsequent differentiation of epithelium into ameloblasts forming enamel does not take place in root formation. (Drawing by John A.M. de Groot)

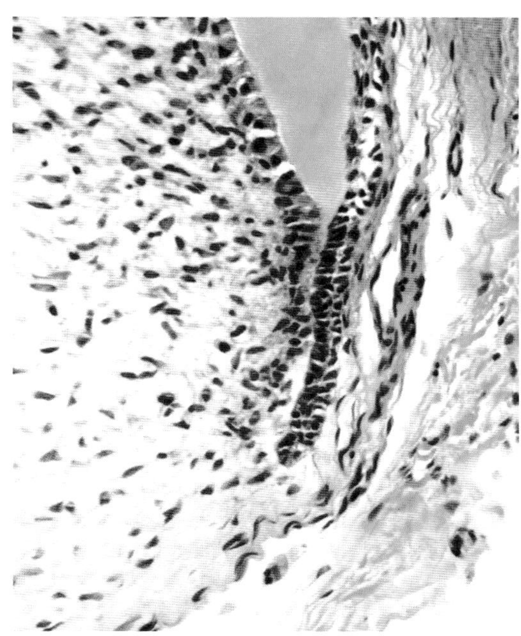

Fig. 1.6 Apical part of tooth germ showing Hertwig's epithelial root sheath. Cylindrical odontoblasts form dentin adjacent to the basal side of the opposing inner enamel epithelium

ity and inhibiting root resorption [2]. Other epithelial reminiscencies to the tooth development lie more superficially in the jaw tissues; they are the epithelial rests of Serres, which originate from the dental lamina.

When the formation of the crown is complete, the enamel organ atrophies. The stellate reticulum disappears and inner and outer enamel epithelium form an epithelial covering of the tooth crown—the so-called reduced enamel epithelium—which remains present until the tooth erupts into the oral cavity. Fluid accumulation between enamel surface and this epithelial investment may give origin to cystic lesions.

In humans, tooth formation starts already at the 6th week of embryonic life. It continues until early adulthood when the roots of the permanent 3rd molars reach their completion. The various stages of tooth development are clearly displayed by jaw radiographs taken from children with a mixed dentition. These radiographs show fully formed deciduous teeth and permanent teeth in varying stages of development. One should realise that all above-described developmental stages may be observed in the jaw at one and the same time as odontogenesis takes place from early embryonic life until early adolescence. To mention just one example, inner and outer enamel epithelium may show active proliferation at the developing root tip while slightly more coronally, the root sheath dissolves and cementoblasts from the dental follicle are lying down cementum, both these events occurring within a distance of only 1 mm from each other at the developing root surface.

References

1. Diekwisch TGH (2001) Developmental biology of cementum. Int J Dev Biol 45:695–706
2. Fujiyama K, Yamashiro T, Fukunaga T et al. (2004) Denervation resulting in dento-alveolar ankylosis associated with decreased Malassez epithelium. J Dent Res 83:625–629
3. Luan X, Ito Y, Diekwisch TGH (2006) Evolution and development of Hertwig's epithelial root sheath. Developmental Dynamics 235:1167–1180
4. Miletich I, Sharpe PT (2004) Neural crest contribution to mammalian tooth formation. Birth Defects Research (Part C) 72:200–212
5. Sharpe PT (2001) Neural crest and tooth morphogenesis. Adv Dent Res 15:4–7
6. Thesleff I, Keränen S, Jernvall J (2001) Enamel knots as signaling centers linking tooth morphogenesis and odontoblast differentiation. Adv Dent Res 15:14–18
7. Tucker A, Sharpe P (2004) The cutting edge of mammalian development. How the embryo makes teeth. Nat Rev Genet 5:499–508
8. Zeichner-David M, Oishi K, Su Z et al. (2003) Role of Hertwig's epithelial root sheath cells in tooth root development. Developmental Dynamics 228:651–663

Chapter 2

Histology of the Teeth and Surrounding Structures

2

2.1 Introduction

Teeth consist for the major part of dentin. This material houses the dental pulp, the soft tissue core of the tooth consisting of myxoid connective tissue with blood vessels and nerves, and supports the enamel cap that covers the part of the tooth that is exposed to the oral cavity. In the root area, dentin is covered by cementum that fixes the collagenous fibres of the periodontal ligament onto the root surface. At the other side, these collagenous fibres are attached to the bone of the tooth socket and in this way, the tooth is fixed in the jaw. Through an opening at the root tip that is called the apical foramen, the connective tissue of the pulp is continuous with the collagenous fibres of the periodontal ligament. Blood vessels and nerves pass through this opening to the dental pulp (Figs. 2.1a, b). Sometimes, additional communications exist between dental pulp and the periodontal ligament. These so-called accessory canals are clinically important as they may cause lesions usually confined to the root tip to occur at aberrant sites.

2.2 Dentin

Dentin is a specialised kind of bone formed by the odontoblasts but different in the sense that it does not contain complete cells but only cellular extensions, i.e., cytoplasmic extensions from the odontoblasts. These cross the full thickness of the dentin from the odontoblastic cell body that lies at the border between dentin and dental pulp to the junction between dentin and enamel. The tiny

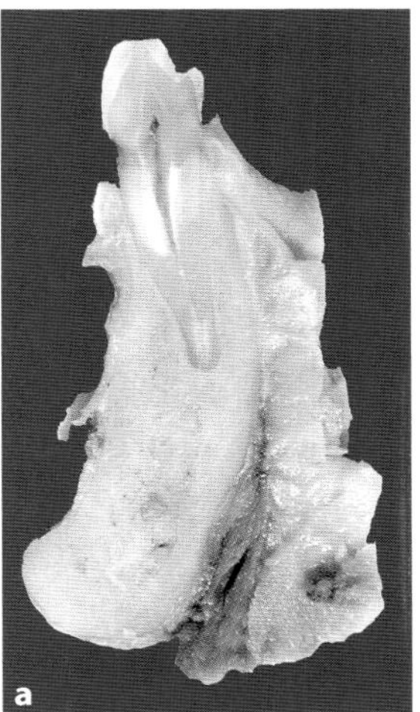

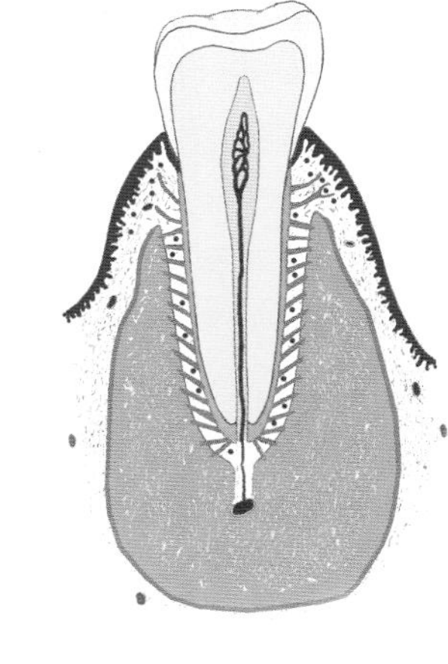

Fig. 2.1 **a** Gross specimen showing tooth in its socket with surrounding jaw bone. **b** Schematic drawing to clarify the various components: enamel in *grey*, dentin in *yellow*, root cementum in *orange*, periodontal ligament in *green* and epithelium in *blue*. (Modified from drawing by John A.M. de Groot)

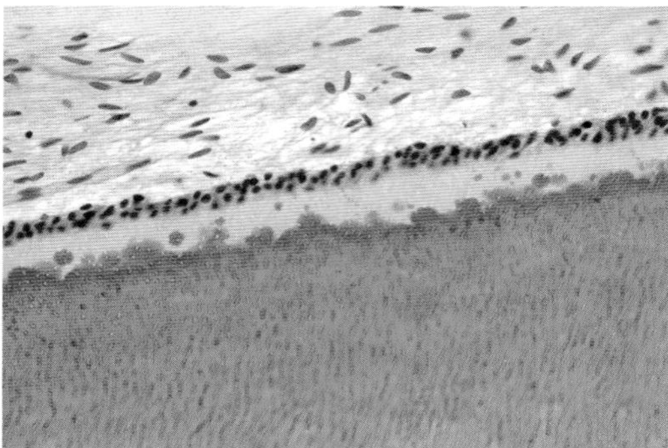

Fig. 2.2 Dentin at its pulpal side bordered by columnar odontoblasts. The distinction between the pale predentin and the darker staining mineralised dentin is clearly visible

canals that house the odontoblastic extensions are recognisable as evenly spaced tubuli. This tubular nature is the histologic hallmark for dentin, not only in teeth but also in odontogenic lesions in which the nature of each mineralised material may not be recognisable at first sight. Sometimes, in the dentin incremental lines that run parallel to the dentino-enamel junction, are observed, the so-called lines of von Ebner.

The organic matrix laid down by the odontoblasts is called predentin; it is recognisable by its pink staining in hematoxylin- and eosin-stained sections. In this matrix, calcification occurs in the form of spherical masses which as they increase in size gradually fuse together, thus transforming the predentin into the darker staining mineralised dentin (Fig. 2.2). At the border between dentin and predentin, these calcospherites can be frequently seen, either separate or already in contact with the calcified dentin.

Several types of dentin are discerned. The layer of dentin immediately adjacent to the border with the enamel is called the mantle dentin. The more centrally located part of the dentin is the circumpulpal dentin. This distinction is relevant as some structural tooth alterations are confined to the circumpulpal dentin, leaving the mantle dentin uninvolved, as will be discussed later on. Mantle dentin is separated from the circumpulpal dentin by a zone of disturbed dentin formation called globular dentin, so-called because of the presence of interglobular spaces due to deficient mineralisation at this site (Figs. 2.3a, b). Both mantle and circumpulpal dentin are taken together as primary dentin. The dentin that is formed during the functional life of the tooth is called secondary dentin. Its life-long gradual deposition causes

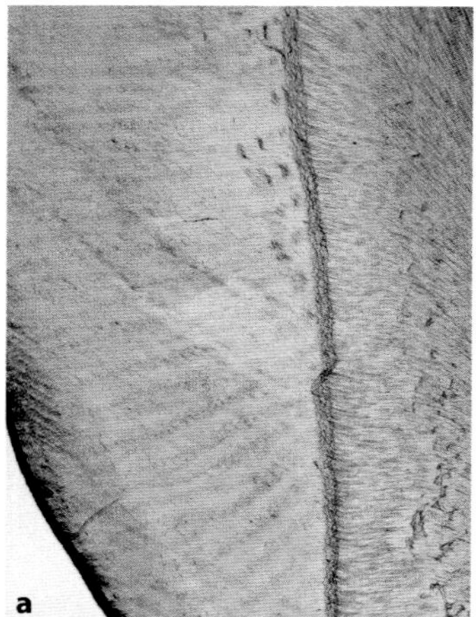

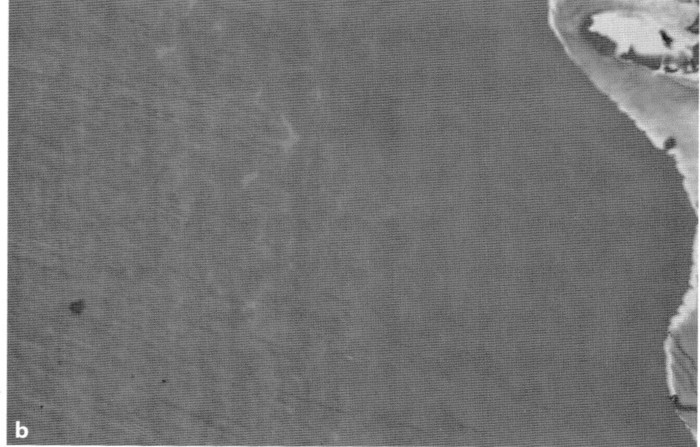

Fig. 2.3 Interglobular dentin recognisable as dark irregularities in an undecalcified ground section, running parallel to the dentino-enamel junction (**a**) or as pale staining areas indicative of incomplete mineralisation in a decalcified hematoxylin- and eosin-stained section (**b**)

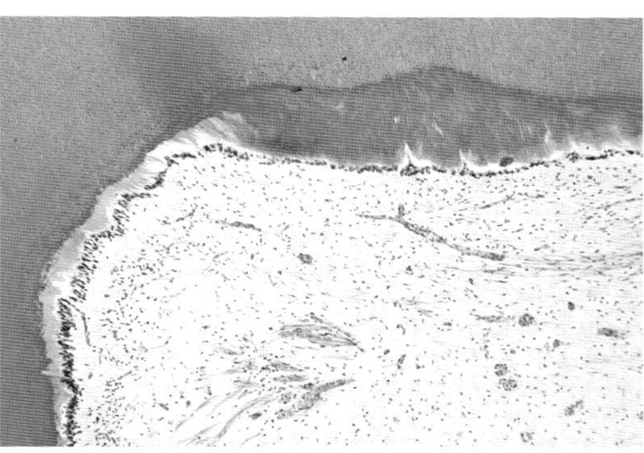

Fig. 2.4 Tertiary dentin shown as an irregular calcified tissue mass interrupting the regular arrangement of odontoblasts

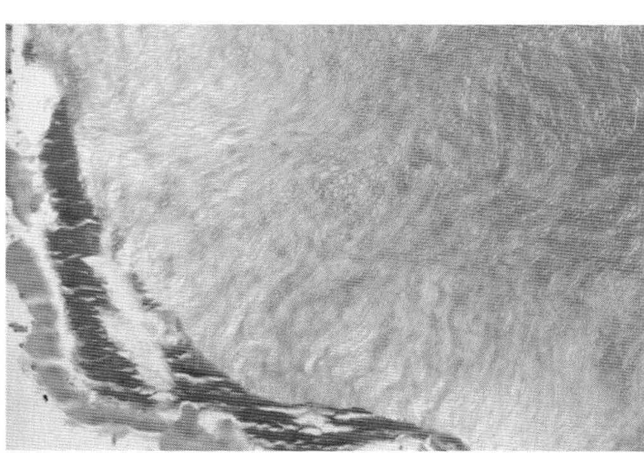

Fig. 2.5 Photomicrograph showing enamel matrix. Due to the low mineral content, its lamellated structure is still visible

a decrease of the pulp chambers over the course of time. Tertiary, or reparative dentin is formed as a pulpal response to some kind of trauma. It differs from both primary and secondary dentin in that it has a more irregular structure, not only containing odontoblastic extensions but also complete cell bodies of odontoblasts and thus resembling bone. That is why it is sometimes also called osteodentin (Fig. 2.4).

Dentin that has lost its organic content due to disappearance of odontoblasts with concomitant disintegration of intratubular cytoplasmic processes is said to contain dead tracts. If these empty tubuli calcify, sclerotic or transparent dentin is formed. Both dead tracts and sclerotic dentin are only visible in undecalcified ground sections.

2.3 Enamel

Enamel content is almost 100% mineral, so it evades histologic evaluation in common paraffin sections from decalcified material. Only in immature tooth tissues, may it be seen in routinely prepared histologic slides due to a still higher proportion of organic components, where it is visible as a slightly basophilic thready material (Fig. 2.5). In this form, it may also form part of the histologic appearance of odontogenic tumours.

Examination of mature enamel requires the employment of ground sections. In transmitted light, incremental lines can be seen in the enamel lying more or less parallel to the crown surface and the dentino-enamel junction, the so-called striae of Retzius. In reflected light, alternating light and dark bands that run perpendicular to the dentino-enamel junction can be observed. These so-called Hunter-Schreger bands are an optical phenomenon caused by different directions of the rods that form the building stones of the enamel (Fig. 2.6). These rods have on transverse

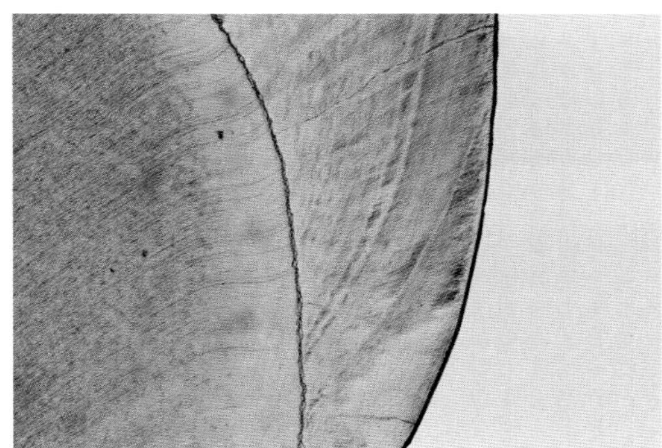

Fig. 2.6 Ground section of a tooth to illustrate in the enamel the presence of the striae of Retzius running parallel to the enamel surface and the alternating light and dark Hunter-Schreger bands running perpendicular to the dentin-enamel junction

sectioning the outline of a keyhole. Through interlocking of these rods, a compact structure is formed. Each rod is formed by four ameloblasts. The rods are responsible for the striated appearance that immature enamel matrix shows in decalcified paraffin sections.

2.4 Cementum

Root cementum is visible as a tiny, slightly basophilic layer at the outer surface of the root part of the tooth and can be distinguished from dentin by the absence of tubuli. It obliterates the peripheral ends of the dentinal tubuli and lies adjacent to the mantle dentin. It is the product of fibroblasts from the dental follicle migrating to the root surface and differentiating into cementoblasts.Whether epithelial cells from Hertwig's sheath contribute to initial cementum formation is controversial as has already been discussed in Chap. 1.

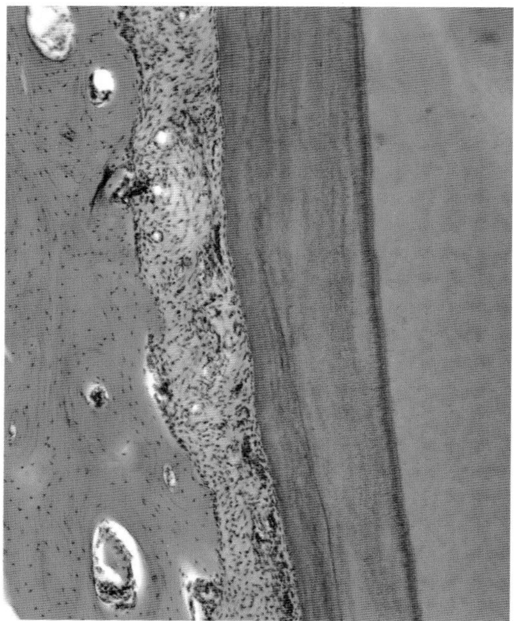

Fig. 2.7 Root surface covered by cementum

Over the course of time, cells from the periodontal ligament may add new cemental layers to the root surface in which cells may become entrapped (Fig. 2.7). The cellular cementum formed in this way closely resembles bone and can only be identified as cementum by its location: covering a root surface. Deposition of cementum probably continues throughout life. It is superimposed upon the cementum that is formed initially during tooth formation. Collagen fibres from the periodontal ligament are embedded in the cementum, thus ensuring fixation of the tooth in its socket. Coronally, cementum ends where enamel starts. Usually, there is a slight overlap, cementum covering the cervical enamel over a short distance. However, an edge-to-edge border as well as a tiny gap between both tooth covering tissues may also be seen.

2.5 Dental Pulp

The dental pulp is the soft connective tissue that forms the inner core of each tooth. It is divided in the coronal part and the radicular part depending on its position. At the root tip, the radicular part of the pulp merges with the periodontal ligament. At this site, blood vessels and nerves enter the tooth. At the interface of pulp and dentin lies a continuous row of columnar odontoblasts (Fig. 2.8). They are responsible for the deposition

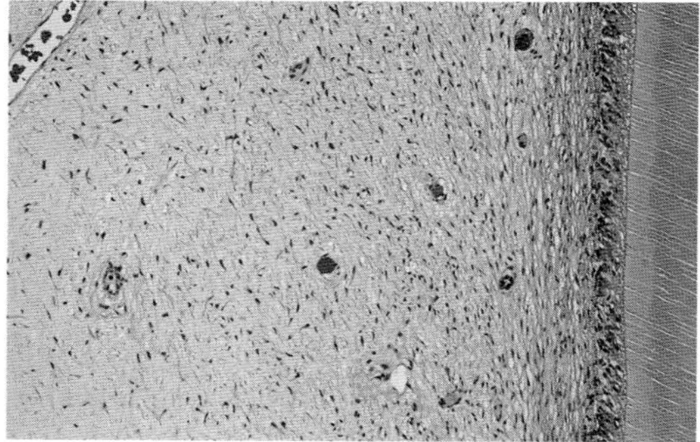

Fig. 2.8 Dental pulp with columnar odontoblasts at the border with the adjacent dentin

of dentinal matrix that may be either secondary as a physiologic process continuing as long as the tooth lives, or tertiary as a reply to some insult. In the latter situation, they lose their regular palissading architecture and may lie embedded in the matrix they have deposited. In the pulp, calcified particles may form, the so-called denticles. They will be discussed more extensively elsewhere (see Sect. 7.1).

2.6 Gingival Attachment

During and after eruption, the tooth pierces through the oral mucosa while reduced enamel epithelium and oral epithelium coalesce (see Chap. 6). To maintain an adequate barrier between the inner and the outer environment, there has to be a firm connection between the epithelial lining of the oral cavity and the surface of the tooth. This requirement is fulfilled by the so-called junctional epithelium, a rim of specialised multilayered nonkeratinising squamous epithelium that forms a cuff attached to and surrounding the necks of the teeth. In a healthy situation, this epithelium is attached to the enamel surface, forming a tapering end at the border between root cementum and enamel. At its opposite end, the junctional epithelium ends in a free margin where it merges with the epithelial surface of the free gingiva, the part of the gingiva that is connected to the tooth surface. This latter epithelium is parakeratinised and shows extremely long and thin rete ridges that may split into several branches. Both the epithelial covering of the free gingiva as well as the junctional epithelium are supported by collagenous fibres fanning out from the root surface and connected to the root through embedding in the root-covering cementum (Figs. 2.9a, b).

The junction between epithelium and tooth is very vulnerable as it depends only on adhesion between both surfaces. Slight inflammatory alterations in the gingiva may already cause disruption of this attachment. The consequences of this disruption will be discussed under the heading gingival and periodontal disease (Chap. 8). Briefly, if there is loss of attachment of the junctional epithelium to the tooth surface, it may move downwards to lie adjacent to the root cementum and may establish a new attachment at that site.

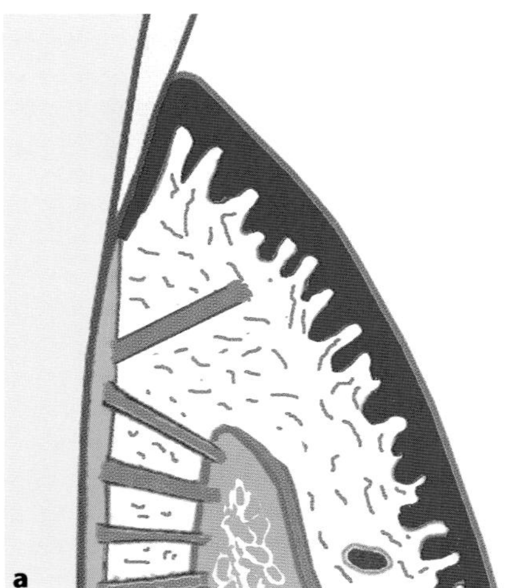

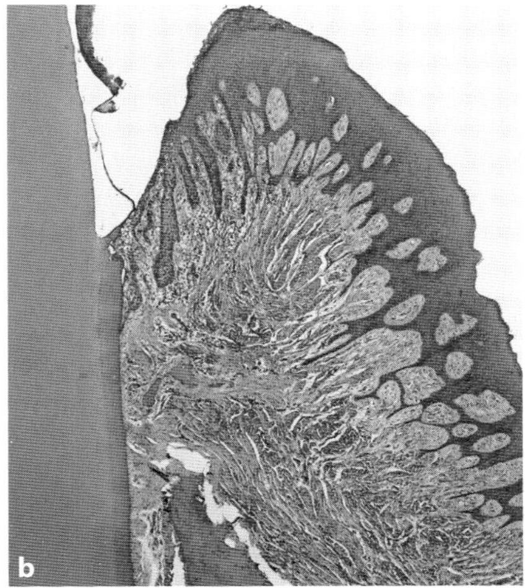

Fig. 2.9 Schematic drawing (**a**) and photomicrograph (**b**) to illustrate the gingival attachment to the tooth surface

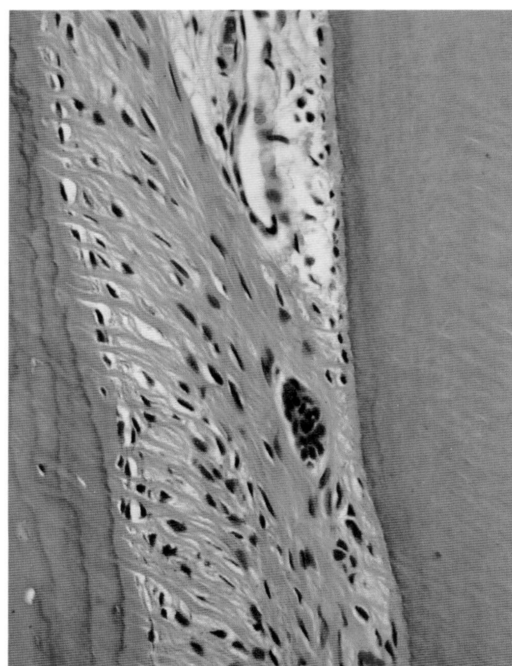

Fig. 2.10 Periodontal ligament, at one side bordered by the bone of the alveolar socket, at the opposite side by the cementum covering the root surface. A nest of Malassez lies embedded between the fibres running between both surfaces

2.7 Periodontal Ligament

When embedded in the jaw in its bony crypt, the tooth is surrounded by a fibrous bag, the so-called dental follicle as has already been mentioned above, and that is not only the source of the periodontal ligament but also for the cells that form the secondary cementum and the alveolar bone.

During and after tooth eruption, the fibrous connective tissue composing the follicle transforms into the periodontal ligament that forms the connection between the tooth and the walls of the bony crypt that evolves into the alveolar socket.

At the neck of the tooth, the dentoalveolar collagenous fibres of the periodontal ligament connect with those of the gingiva, which are specifically known as gingival fibres. Epithelial rests of Malassez, already mentioned before, lie embedded in the collagen fibres between alveolar bone and root surface (Fig. 2.10).

The dental follicle is extremely important from a differential diagnostic point of view. It may contain structures that are also found in a variety of odontogenic tumours and that may be mistaken as proof for presence of such a tumour by the unaware pathologist. This point will be discussed more extensively within the context of odontogenic tumours (see Chaps. 10 and 11).

Further reading

Avery JK, Chiego DJ Jr. (2006) Essentials of oral histology and embryology. A clinical approach, 3rd edn. Mosby-Elsevier. St. Louis

Chapter 3

Disturbed Tooth Form

3

3.1 Disturbances Arising During Tooth Formation

Teeth may show an abnormal form due to malformations occurring during development or acquired after eruption into the oral cavity. The microscopic structure of the dental tissues usually is normal.

3.1.1 Fusion

In case of fusion, two adjacent teeth are connected with each other by either enamel and dentin both or, rarely, by enamel alone. The fusion may be complete over the full length of the teeth or only partial. The condition is due to the merging of two adjacent tooth germs. If the tooth germs touch each other after the investing dental follicle has disappeared, odontogenic soft tissues may unite to form a common matrix that subsequently mineralises as usual (Figs. 3.1a–e). The number of teeth will be diminished by one in this condition, two normal teeth being replaced by one of abnormal appearance. Theoretically, the dentition can still have a normal number of teeth when there is fusion of a tooth with a supernumerary counterpart. Occurrence of a separate dentin stalk projecting from the root surface and capped with enamel and having a common pulp chamber with the main tooth probably represents this type of fusion.

3.1.2 Gemination and Twinning

Gemination occurs when there is partial development of two teeth from one single tooth germ. An abnormally formed tooth with usually one root canal is the outcome of this developmental fault (Figs. 3.2a, b). When the division is complete, the condition is called twinning. Then, the normal number of teeth is increased by one, the superfluous tooth usually being the mirror image of its adjacent counterpart. As already mentioned, the distinction between gemination and fusion is made by counting the number of teeth in the dentition. In case of fusion, their number is decreased by one as two teeth are replaced by one single abnormally formed fusion product. In case of gemination, the number is normal but with one of the teeth being replaced by an abnormally formed one.

3.1.3 Concrescence

Concrescence is the connection of two or more teeth by root cementum alone after the tooth crowns have been formed (Figs. 3.3a–d). The teeth themselves are usually normal of size and form. As the uniting tissue is cementum, an increased amount of cementum covering the roots—hypercementosis—is usually also present.

3.1.4 Dens Invaginatus

Dens invaginatus, also called dens in dente, is a condition in which the crown surface of the tooth invaginates deeply into the crown and quite often also the root part. In this way, a deep groove is created, lined by dentin with a thin surface layer of enamel. Externally, the involved tooth may only show a tiny pit at its outer surface. In the interior of the tooth, this pit dilates to form a large cavity (Figs. 3.4a–d). Through this pit, baca

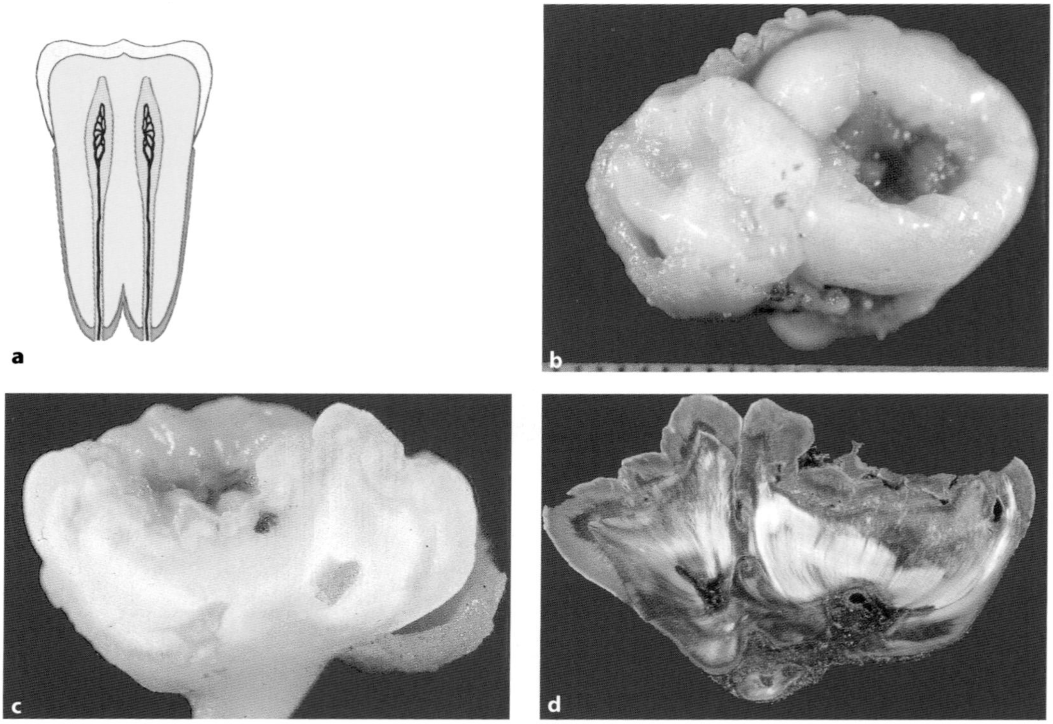

b

c

d

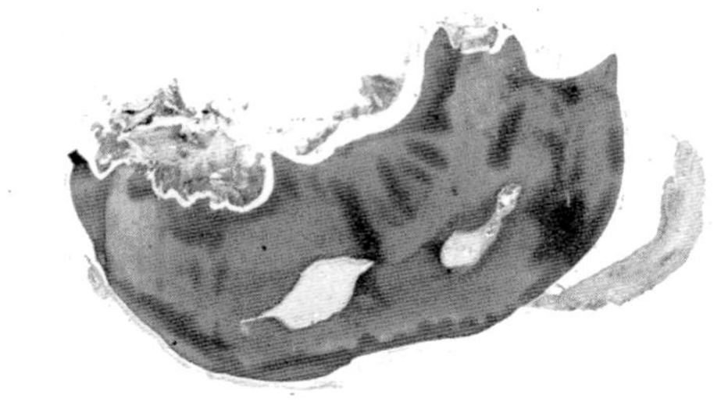

e

Fig. 3.1 Schematic drawing (**a**), gross appearance (**b**), cut surface (**c**), ground section (**d**), and decalcified section (**e**) of fusion. Two teeth are connected to each other at the level of the dentin, indicating contact between two teeth during their germ stage

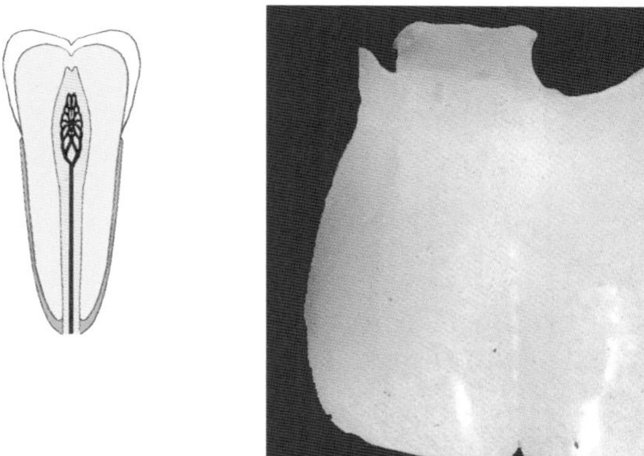

Fig. 3.2 Schematic drawing (**a**) and gross appearance (**b**) of gemination

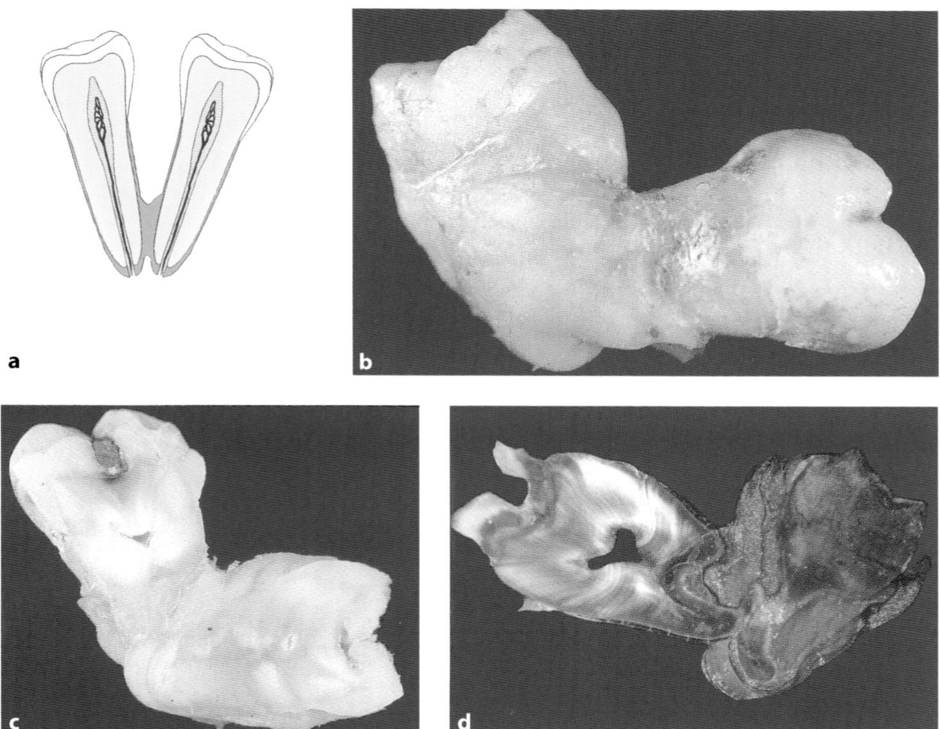

Fig. 3.3a–d Schematic drawing (**a**) and gross appearance (**b**), cut surface (**c**), and ground section (**d**) of concrescence. Two teeth are united by a thick cementum layer

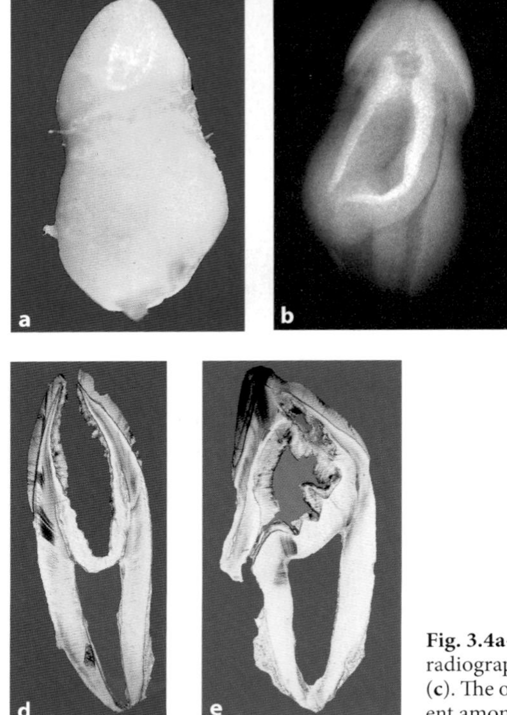

Fig. 3.4a–e Dens invaginatus (dens in dente). Gross appearance (**a**), radiograph (**b**) and cut surface to display the cavity inside the tooth (**c**). The opening of the invagination to the outer surface may be different among individual cases: **d** incisally, **e** laterally

teria from the oral environment have free access to the inner part of the tooth and therefore, this form anomaly makes these teeth very vulnerable for carious decay. The outer opening of the invagination may also be located laterally (Fig. 3.4e).

3.1.5 Dens Evaginatus

In dens evaginatus, an enamel-covered tubercle projects from the occlusal surface of the affected tooth. This evagination not only consists of enamel but also of dentin and pulp tissue. It mostly occurs in molar and premolar teeth (Fig. 3.5).

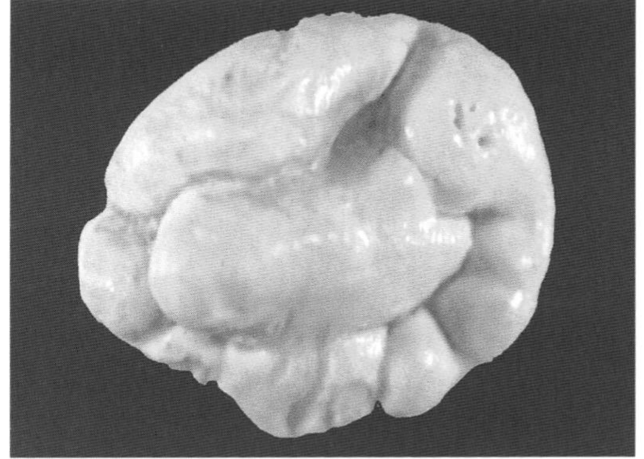

Fig. 3.5 Dens evaginatus. The occlusal surface of the molar tooth shows a centrally located additional cusp

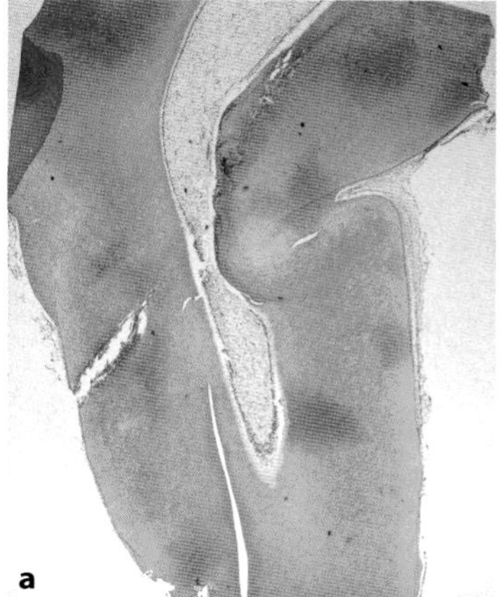

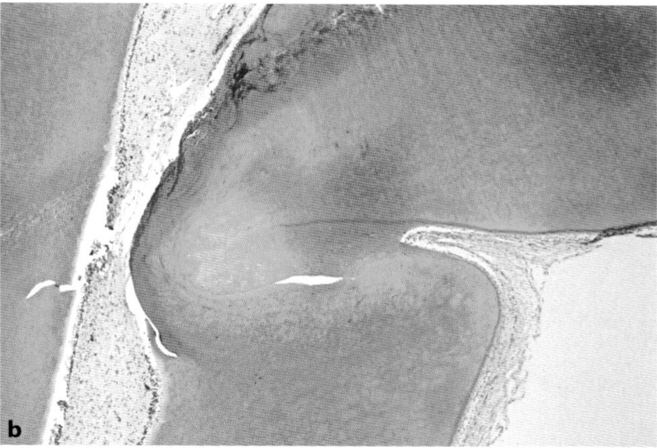

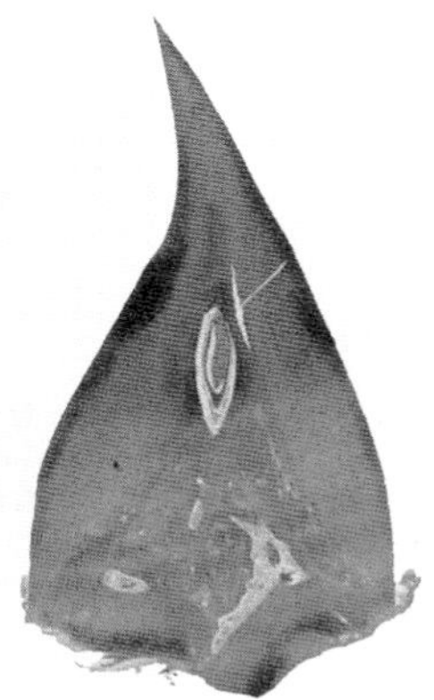

Fig. 3.6a–c Dilaceration. The root shows an acute angle (**a**). At higher magnification, the disturbed course of the dentinal tubuli is shown (**b**). Sometimes, the entire root is stunted and underdeveloped (**c**)

3.1.6 Dilaceration

Dilaceration means displacement of the crown from its normal alignment with the root. It occurs when during tooth development an acute mechanical event causes a movement of the already calcified coronal part of the tooth germ that is not adequately followed by the not-yet-calcified root part of the tooth. In this way, a persistent malalignment between both components will be established, the root forming an angle with the crown in the adult tooth; alternatively only a stunted root may be formed (Figs. 3.6a–c). Malformation of the immature tooth may also occur through forces exerted by intraosseous space-occupying lesions. In those cases, the teeth involved show bending and no angulation. This type of malformation is not included in the definition of dilaceration.

3.1.7 Taurodontism

In normal teeth, the pulp chamber shows a constriction at the level of the amelocemental junction. In taurodontism, the pulp chamber shows an increased vertical dimension, thus extending far into the root area of the involved tooth. As a consequence, in multirooted teeth, the splitting of the root into its several extensions, the so-called

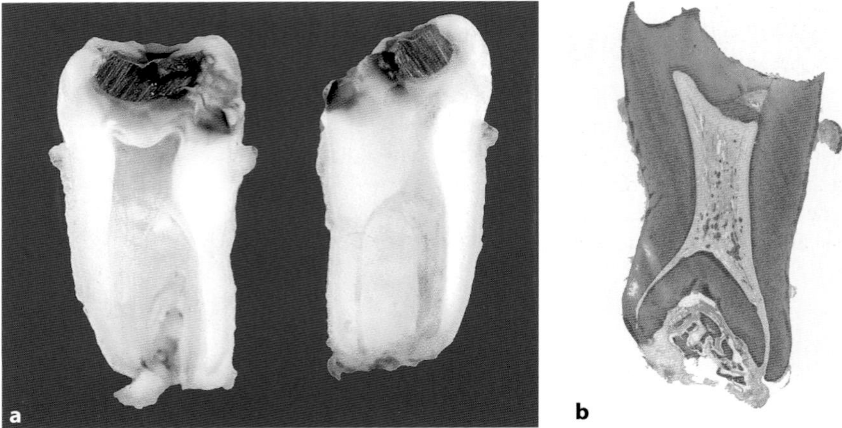

Fig. 3.7 Cut surface (**a**) and histologic appearance (**b**) of taurodontism. The apical displacement of the root furcation is clearly visible

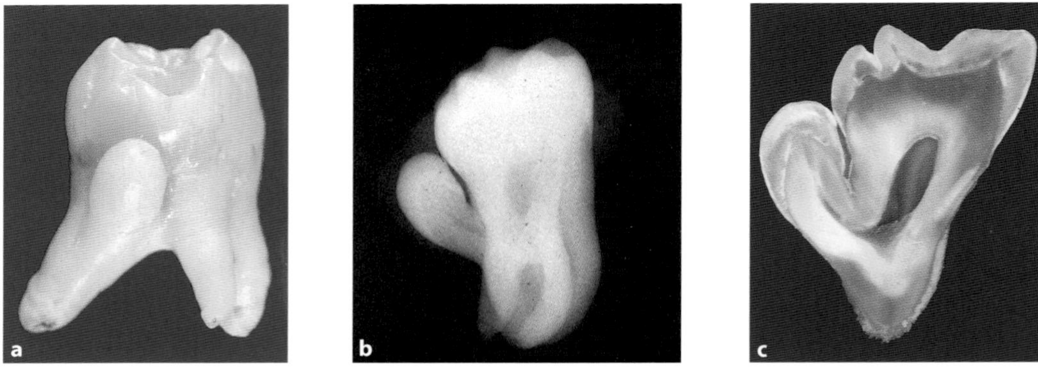

Fig. 3.8 Gross appearance (**a**), radiograph (**b**), and ground section (**c**) of an enamel-capped lateral outgrowth from the root surface. This could be classified as an enamel pearl although fusion of the molar tooth with a rudimentary supernumerary tooth could also be considered

furcation, occurs at a level much more apically than is the case in normal teeth (Figs. 3.7a, b). Therefore, the root bi- or trifurcation may be very shallow or even absent.

3.1.8 Enamel Pearls

Enamel pearls are deposits of enamel in an abnormal position, mostly the outer root surface, although they can also be found embedded in the dentin. Their size may vary from a pinpoint to several millimeters. Sometimes, the enamel pearl has the form of a cap covering a dome-shaped dentin core. If this type of enamel pearl has a considerable size, its distinction from a supernumerary tooth fused becomes debatable (Figs. 3.8a–c).

3.2 Posteruptively Acquired Disturbed Tooth Form

After their eruption in the oral cavity, teeth may undergo form alterations due to trauma causing loss of tooth substance due to fractures. Also, tooth substance may be lost gradually due to carious decay. Both issues and their sequelae will be discussed in Chap. 5.

Further reading

Tahmassebi JF, Day PF, Toumba J et al. (2003) Paediatric dentistry in the new millennium: 6. Dental anomalies in children. Dental Update 30:534–540

Chapter 4

Developmental Disturbances in Tissue Structure

4

4.1 Enamel

As enamel content is almost 100% mineral, it cannot withstand the decalcification needed to allow paraffin sectioning. Therefore, in general, it is not present anymore in the histologic sections and so, the histopathologist usually will not be faced with problems of how to interpret changes in this tissue type. However, as gross inspection of submitted teeth before they are processed for histology will already yield useful data, alterations in this dental hard tissue will nevertheless be mentioned briefly from a practical point of view while acknowledging that the topic is much more complicated then depicted below.

4.1.1 Amelogenesis Imperfecta

Amelogenesis imperfecta is a hereditary condition afflicting the tooth enamel. It is subdivided in a considerable number of conditions depending on the clinical appearance, the kind of disturbance, and the pattern of inheritance which may be autosomal recessive, autosomal dominant, or x-linked. For practical purposes, amelogenesis imperfecta will be discussed to allow recognition of the various subtypes as defined by their gross appearance, teeth either showing abnormal enamel caps of normal hardness or enamel caps consisting of enamel that is too soft and discolored. The first is called hypoplastic, and the latter hypomineralised or hypomatured. The ambiguities arising from this phenotypic classification are demonstrated by the combined occurrence of both hypoplastic and hypomineralised amelogenesis imperfecta in a family also having taurodontism [14] and it has been proposed recently that a classification based on the mode of inheritance may be more appropriate [1]. The current description aims to provide a practically applicable guide.

As amelogenesis is a hereditary condition, it afflicts in principle all teeth or nearly all teeth, although there may be variation in expression.

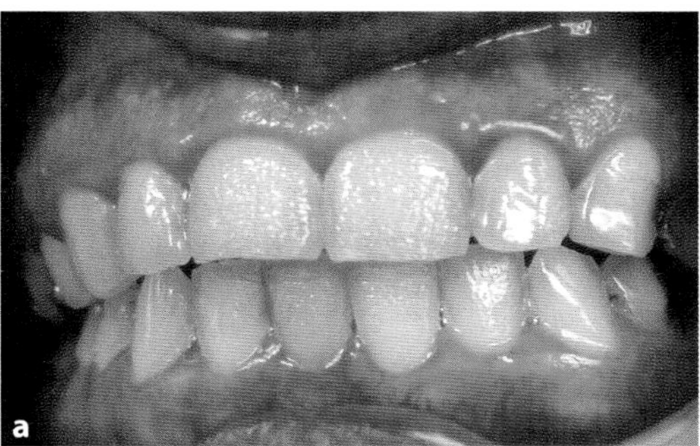

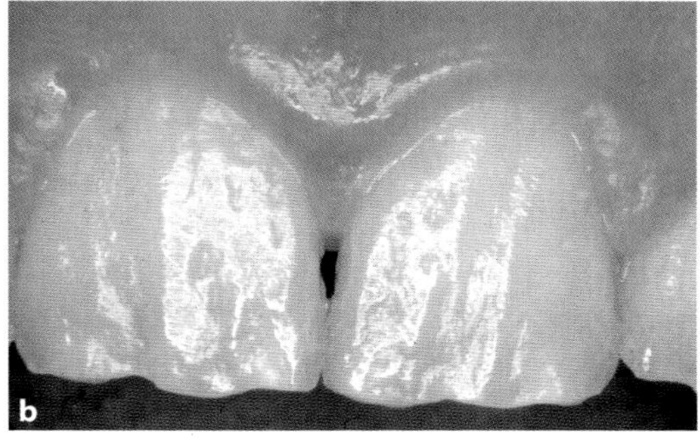

Fig. 4.1a,b Amelogenesis imperfecta of the hypoplastic type. Tooth surface shows pitting (**a**) or irregularities (**b**) indicating abnormal enamel formation. The hardness of the enamel is normal

4.1.1.1 Amelogenesis Imperfecta, Hypoplastic

Amelogenesis imperfecta of the hypoplastic type is the result of a decreased amount of enamel matrix laid down during tooth formation. As a result, the enamel cap does not acquire its normal thickness. As mineralisation is normal, the hardness of the remaining enamel layer may be normal. However, the reduced thickness of the enamel cap causes an abnormal crown form of the involved teeth. These externally visible abnormalities may vary from an almost absent enamel cap to only a few irregularities in an otherwise normally formed tooth. These irregularities have been classified as rough, pitted, and grooves that may run vertically or horizontally (Figs. 4.1a, b).

4.1.1.2 Amelogenesis Imperfecta, Hypomineralised

In the hypomineralised type of amelogenesis imperfecta, the enamel initially develops a normal thickness but the matrix is not mineralised in a normal way. Therefore, the teeth erupt with an initially normal appearance of their crowns but the ill-mineralised enamel is soft and as a result, is easily worn away in the mechanically demanding oral environment, thus exposing the underlying

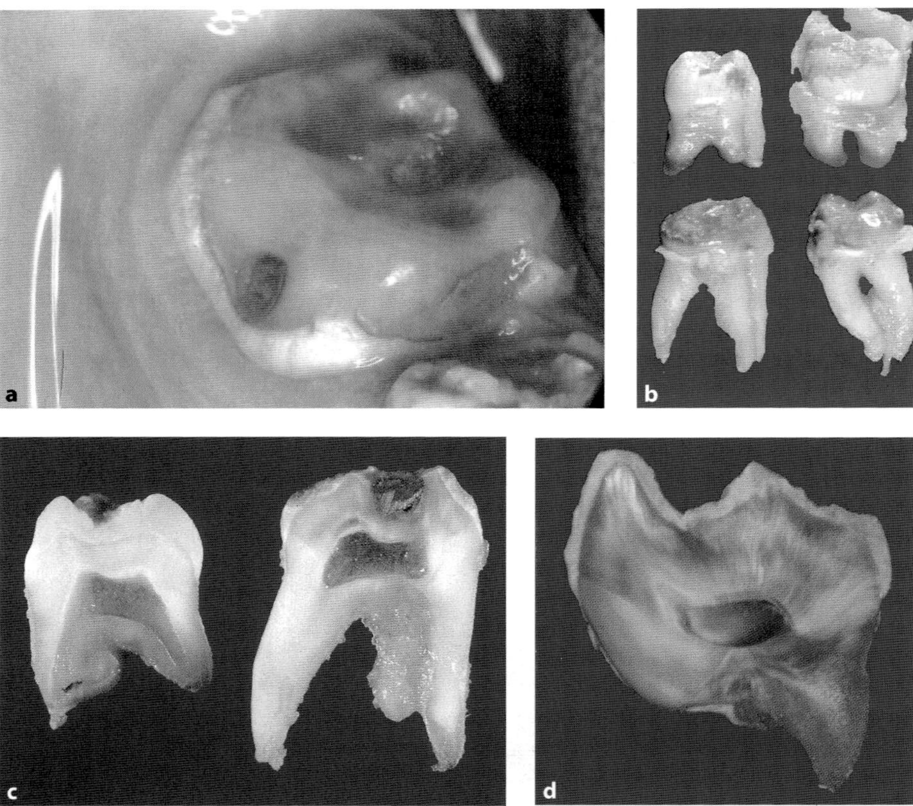

Fig. 4.2a–d Amelogenesis imperfecta of the hypomineralised type. The enamel cap is worn away due to masticatory forces leaving a bare dentin surface with enamel remnants present only at the cervical part of the crown (**a**). Gross appearance (**b**), cut surface (**c**) and ground section (**d**) showing thin and friable enamel cap

dentin. The enamel is light yellow-brown to orange and becomes brown to black after eruption because of stains from food or beverages. Characteristically, remnants of enamel remain present in mechanically privileged niches, e.g., the cervical part of the tooth crown (Figs. 4.2a–d). Due to its low content of minerals, this defective enamel will not dissolve completely during decalcification and therefore, it may be present in paraffin sections made from these teeth (Fig. 4.3).

4.1.1.3 Amelogenesis Imperfecta, Hypomatured

Amelogenesis of the hypomatured type is difficult to discern from the hypomineralised type as it also shows the presence of enamel that is softer than it should be and that shows discoloration.

4.1.2 Enamel Hypoplasia

Enamel hypoplasia means any disturbance in tooth formation leading to macroscopically visible defects in the surface of the enamel. Although this definition also would include the hypoplastic form of amelogenesis imperfecta, the term enamel hypoplasia in practice is only applied to enamel lesions due to a systemic interference. This means that alterations may not be universal in the sense that they involve all teeth or the entire teeth crown, as is the case in amelogenesis imperfecta. Only the enamel formed during the time span in which the systemic interfering factor was active will be abnormal. As the enamel is lost during decalcification, microscopy of this form of abnormal enamel requires ground sections, which is not within the reach of most histopathology laboratories. However, macroscopical inspection of these teeth will allow the distinction from amelogenesis imperfecta, where all teeth show abnormalities, as opposed to enamel hypoplasia, where only some teeth may be abnormal. A common cause for enamel hypoplasia is an overdose of fluoride. This condition will be discussed more extensively below. Also tetracyclin may give rise to enamel hypoplasia, but as these drugs particularly cause tooth pigmentation, this topic will be discussed under that heading.

4.1.3 Enamel Opacities

Enamel opacities are white opaque spots in smooth-surfaced enamel. Probably they are due to transient hypomineralisation of the enamel matrix. Most often, they are seen at the incisor teeth (Fig. 4.4). Incidentally, they may also be

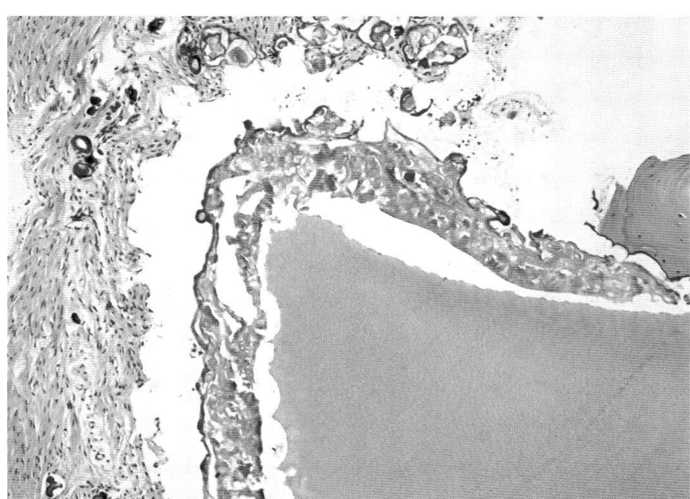

Fig. 4.3 Sometimes, teeth are covered by a defective enamel layer displaying both features of hypoplasia and hypomineralisation as shown in this photomicrograph. The enamel layer shows variation in thickness and absence of regular lamellation (compare with Fig. 2.5). Underlying dentin does not show any abnormalities

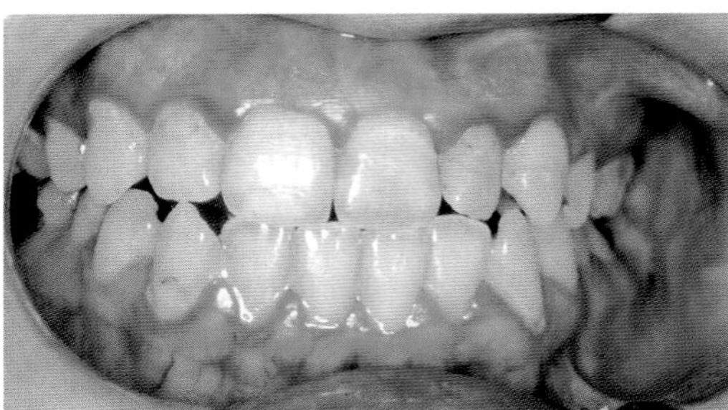

Fig. 4.4 White spot on labial surface of right first incisor tooth indicates transient period of hypocalcification

brown and mottled. In that case, distinction from local enamel hypoplasia may become equivocal. The prevalence of this condition is rather high. Enamel opacities are probably the result of short intervals of disturbed deposition of enamel matrix. Subsequent normal formation of enamel matrix will then bury the abnormal area.

4.1.4 Dental Fluorosis

Fluorosis is a permanent hypomineralisation of enamel, in its mildest form characterised as small white spots. More severe forms range between white, opaque areas to darkly stained and pitted enamel (Figs. 4.5a, b). Probably, an overdose of fluoride interferes both with the function of ameloblasts and proper calcification of the enamel matrix [10, 13].

4.2 Dentin

Structural abnormalities of dentin, quite often also resulting in abnormally formed teeth, mostly have an hereditary background. They are classified into two main groups: dentinogenesis imperfecta and dentinal dysplasia. Dentinogenesis imperfecta is further subdivided: type I, occurring together with osteogenesis imperfecta; and type II, occurring isolated. Dentinal dysplasia is also subdivided into two types. All types are characterised by failure of normal dentin formation after the initial deposition of a small amount of mantle dentin. As a result of this, involved teeth may show either abnormally short or entirely absent roots, whereas the pulpal chambers may partly or entirely obliterated due to formation of abnormal dentin masses. When dentin apposition comes to a halt almost immediately after it has started, rootless teeth with a very thin dentin cap are the result: the so-called shell-teeth. Due to overlapping phenotypes for all clinical categories of heritable dentin defects, their categorisation has been extensively discussed in the past and it has been proposed recently that a classification based on the underlying genetic defect should replace the phenotypic classification [3, 6–8, 11, 12].

For the histopathologist, the heritable dentin defects are recognisable by the presence of a small rim of normal dentin covering either an unusually wide pulp space in shell teeth or encasing a pulp chamber filled with irregular masses of dentin containing haphazardly running dentinal tubuli

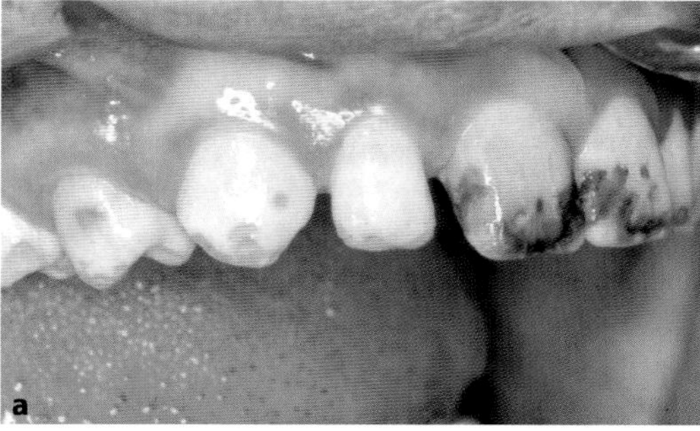

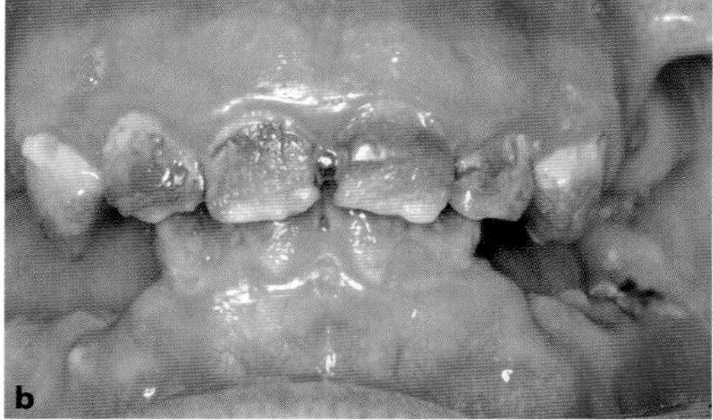

Fig. 4.5 Dental fluorosis. The abnormalities may vary from moderate (**a**) to severe (**b**). Enamel shows white spots, brown discolorations, and surface irregularities indicating both enamel hypocalcification and hypomineralisation

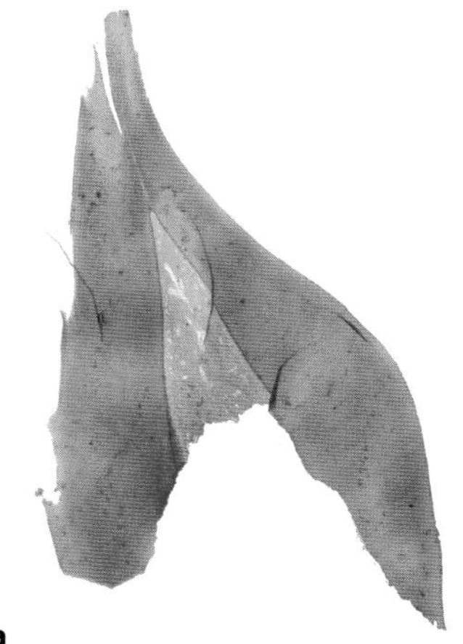

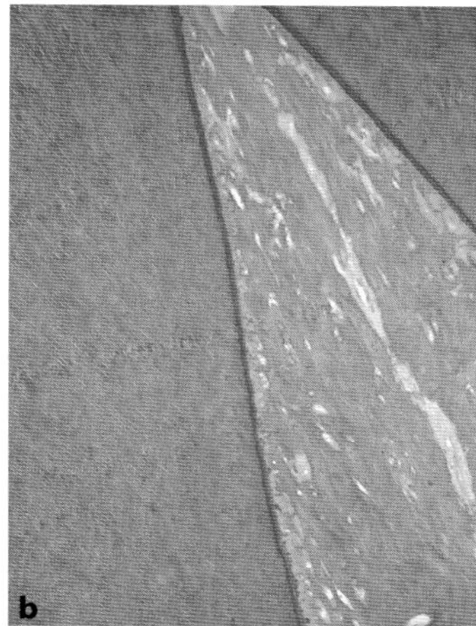

Fig. 4.6 Tooth showing thin surface layer of regular dentin and pulpal obliteration by irregular dentinal masses (**a**) with vascular inclusions (**b**). This appearance may be shown by both dentinogenesis imperfecta as well as dentinal dysplasia

in the other categories (Figs. 4.6a, b). This abnormal dentin should not be confused with the tertiary dentin formed locally in the dental pulp as a response to some external irritant (see Chap. 5).

4.3 Developmental Structural Abnormalities Involving Both Enamel and Dentin

4.3.1 Odontodysplasia

Odontodysplasia is a developmental disturbance consisting of both enamel and dentin abnormalities in several adjacent teeth. The often-added suffix "regional" emphasises this usually localised character, but a few cases have been described with involvement of more extensive parts of the dentition, the abnormal teeth being present bilaterally and in both upper and lower jaw. The teeth are abnormally formed and the covering enamel layer is thin and yellow. The pulp chambers are wide and the amount of dentin is greatly reduced. The enamel is hypoplastic and the dentin contains large areas of interglobular dentin (Figs. 4.7a, b). Also, the predentin zone is very wide. The dental pulp usually contains large and irregular aggregates of mineralised matrix, the so-called denticles (see Chap. 7). The condition may be accompanied by gingival enlargement [4, 5].

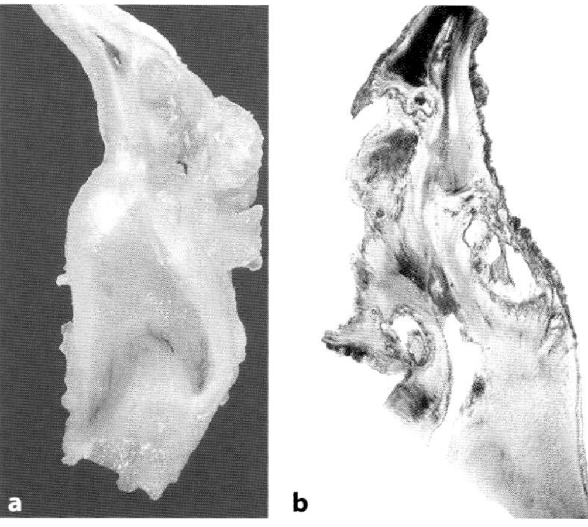

Fig. 4.7 Cut surface (**a**) and ground section (**b**) from tooth showing features of odontodysplasia. Both enamel and dentin are abnormal

4.3.2 Odontogenesis Imperfecta

In odontogenesis imperfecta, both enamel and dentin exhibit pathologic changes in all teeth. The enamel is hypoplastic and the dentin shows changes similar to those seen in dentinogenesis imperfecta (Figs. 4.8a, b).

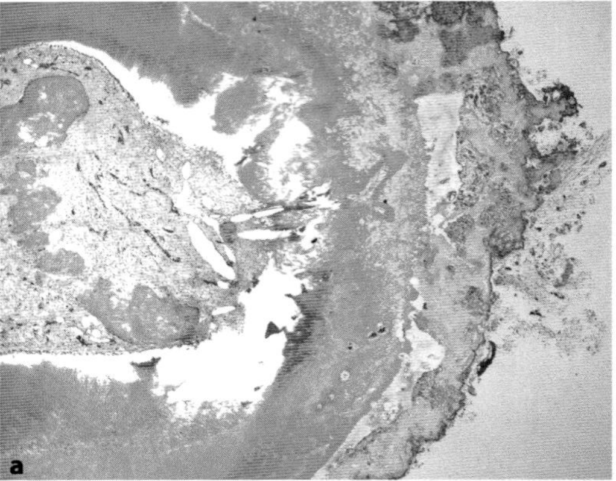

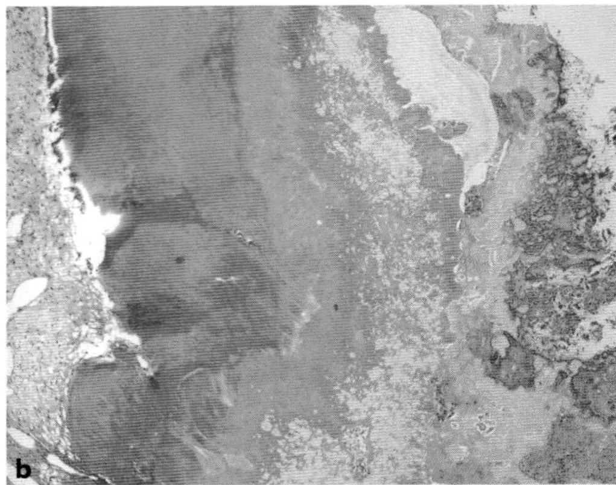

Fig. 4.8 Low power view (**a**) and higher magnification (**b**) indicating both abnormal dentin as well as enamel. The dentin is thin and contains vascular inclusions and the enamel lacks lamellation and shows uneven mineralisation. This pattern indicates disturbances of both enamel as well as dentin formation and could be indicative of odontodysplasia as well as odontogenesis imperfecta depending on the distribution among the dentition

4.3.3 Rickets

Lack of adequate supply of vitamin D during tooth development results in enamel hypoplasia (Fig. 4.9). Changes in the dentin especially are apparent in cases of vitamin D-resistant rickets (hereditary hypophosphataemia). This condition is associated with the presence of large pulp chambers, pronounced interglobular dentin, wide seams of predentin and clefts, and tubular defects in the dentin formed in areas of tapering pulpal extensions (Fig. 4.10).

4.3.4 Segmental Odontomaxillary Dysplasia

Segmental odontomaxillary dysplasia is a rare, unilateral developmental disorder of the maxilla involving abnormal growth and maturation of the bone, lack of one or both premolars, altered primary molar structure, delayed tooth eruption, and fibrous hyperplasia of the gingiva (Fig. 4.11). Data on histology of the involved teeth are scarce, only one report mentioning them. These authors report the presence of tubular defects

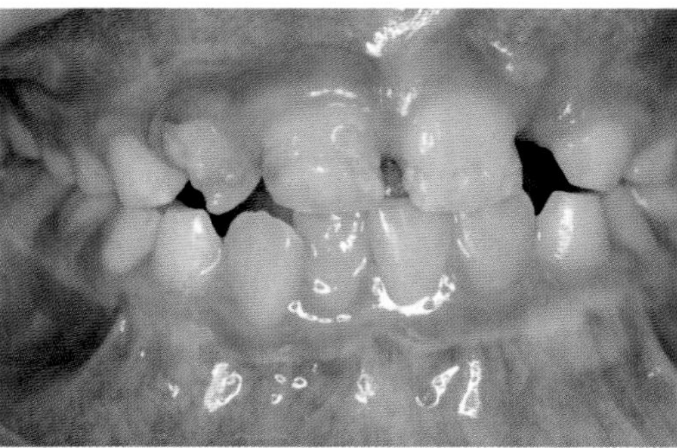

Fig. 4.9 Dentition showing irregular surfaces of various teeth due to defective enamel formation caused by rickets

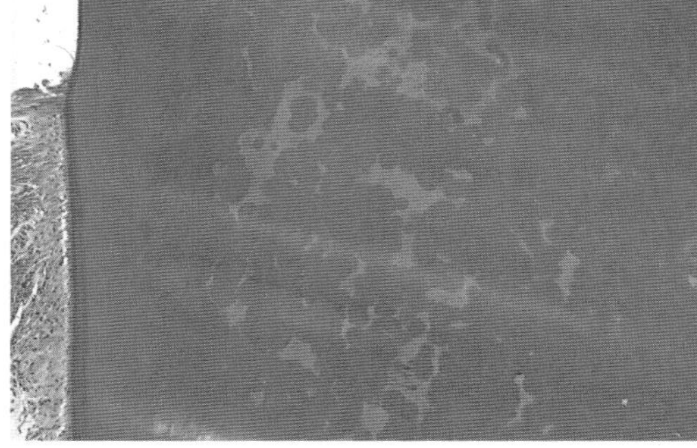

Fig. 4.10 Photomicrograph showing excessive interglobular dentin due to defective mineralisation in hereditary hypophosphataemia

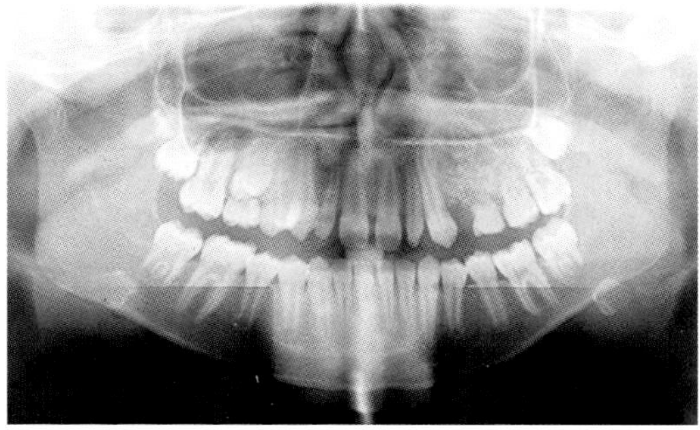

Fig. 4.11 Segmental odontomaxillary dysplasia. X-ray showing area of irregular bone structure in left maxilla. Two teeth in this area show an abnormal root contour indicating resorption

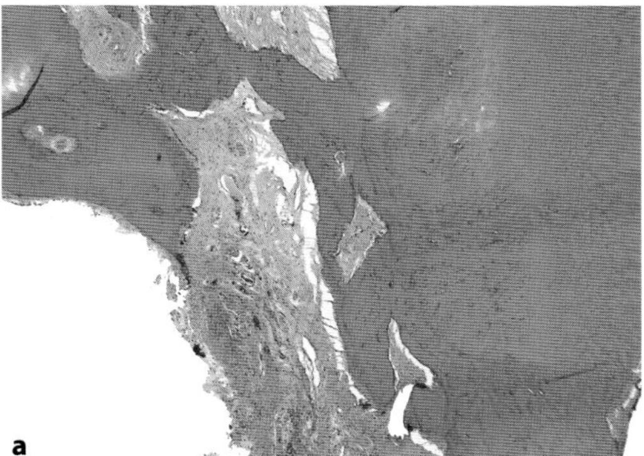

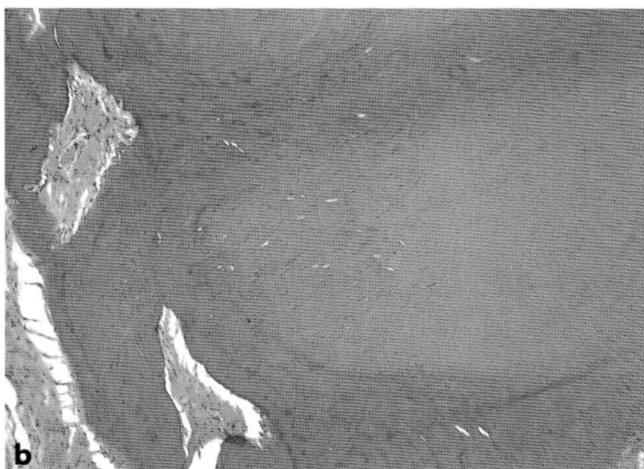

Fig. 4.12 Teeth in segmental odontomaxillary dysplasia show pulp fibrosis, lack of an odontoblastic layer, and an irregular architecture of the circumpulpal dentin (**a**). This dentin shows haphazardly running tubuli and cellular inclusions. The outer part of the dentin (**b**,) is normal

in the coronal dentin extending from the pulp towards the dentino-enamel junction. The circumpulpal dentin from the middle one-third of the root apically had an irregular tubular structure and lacked a well-defined odontoblast layer (Figs. 4.12a, b). The pulp chamber had an irregular outline, giving the impression of intradentinal pulpal inclusions with pulp stones. Pulp chamber and root canals were enlarged. Pulpal tissues showed coarse fibrosis, increased vascularity, and a whorled pattern. External root surfaces showed areas of resorption, some of them with partial repair [2, 9].

References

1. Aldred MJ, Savarirayan R, Crawford PJM (2003) Amelogenesis imperfecta: a classification and catalogue for the 21st century. Oral Diseases 9:19–23
2. Armstrong C, Napier SS, Boyd RC et al. (2004) Case report. Histopathology of the teeth in segmental odontomaxillary dysplasia. New findings. J Oral Pathol Med 33:246–248
3. Beattie ML, Kim JW, Gong SG et al. (2006) Phenotypic variation in dentinogenesis imperfecta/dentin dysplasia linked to 4q21. J Dent Res 85:329–333
4. Crawford PJM, Aldred MJ (1989) Regional odontodysplasia: a bibliography. J Oral Pathol 18:251–263

5. Fanibunda KB, Voames JV (1996) Odontodysplasia, gingival manifestations, and accompanying abnormalities. Oral Surg Oral Med Oral Pathol Oral Radiol Endod 81:84–88
6. MacDougall M (2003) Dental structural diseases mapping to human chromosome 4q21. Connect Tissue Res. 44 Suppl 1:285–291
7. O'Carrol MK, Duncan WK, Perkins TM (1991) Dentin dysplasia: review of the literature and a proposed subclassificiation based on radiographic findings. Oral Surg Oral Med Oral Pathol 72:119–125
8. Parekh S, Kyriazidou A, Bloch-Zupan A et al. (2006) Multiple pulp stones and shortened roots of unknown etiology. Oral Surg Oral Med Oral Pathol Oral Radiol Endod 101:e139–e142
9. Prusack N, Pringle G, Scotti V et al. (2000) Segmental odontomaxillary dysplasia. A case report and review of the literature. Oral Surg Oral Med Oral Pathol Oral Radiol Endod 90:483–888
10. Robinson C, Connell S, Kirkham J et al. (2004) The effect of fluoride on the developing tooth. Caries Res 38:268–276
11. Shields ED, Bixler D, El-Kafraway (1973) A proposed classification for heritable human dentine defects with a description of a new entity. Arch Oral Biol 18:543–553
12. Steidler NE, Radden BG, Reade PC (1984) Dentinal dysplasia. A clinicopathological study of eight cases and review of the literature. Br J Oral Maxillofac Surg 22:274–286.
13. Tahmassebi JF, Day PF, Toumba J et al. (2003) Paediatric dentistry in the new millennium: 6. Dental anomalies in children. Dental Update 30:534–540
14. Witkop CJ Jr (1988) Amelogenesis imperfecta, dentinogenesis imperfecta and dentin dysplasia revisited: problems in classification. J Oral Pathol 17:547–553

Chapter 5

Alterations Acquired After Tooth Eruption

5

Tooth alterations occurring after eruption in the oral cavity are manifold. They may be due to a large variety of causes. Their effects may be gross form alterations or subtle changes only visible on histologic examination.

5.1 Caries

Tooth decay (dental caries) starts with the destruction of the enamel cap by micro-organisms present in the oral cavity and adherent to the tooth surface. This leads to exposure of the underlying dentin to the oral environment and to its destruction by bacterial proteolytic enzymes. Enamel caries will not be visible in routinely prepared histologic sections as this tissue dissolves completely during decalcification. In ground sections made from undecalcified teeth, microscopic examination under transmitted light will reveal optical alterations related to decreased mineral content of a still-intact crystalline structure. These alterations tend to occur over a cone-shaped area having its base on the surface and its point towards the amelo-dentinal junction (Fig. 5.1). With increasing loss of minerals from the enamel structure, this tissue will disintegrate. Sometimes, this destroyed enamel will contain so much organic material that it is still present in decalcified sections where it is visible as a basophilic amorphous mass.

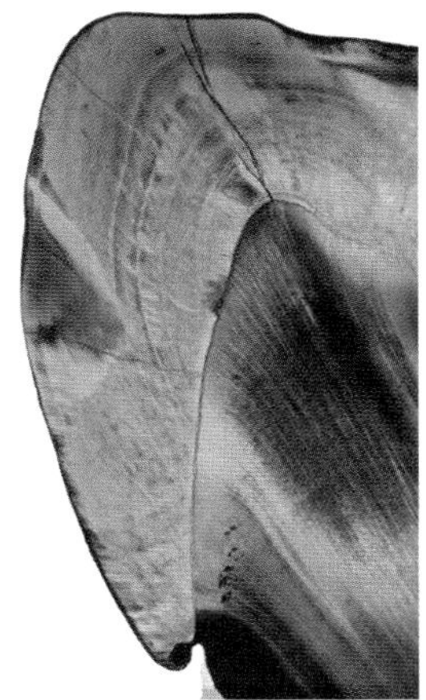

Fig. 5.1 Ground section showing wedge-shaped discoloration in enamel due to alterations in optical properties of enamel as a result of loss of calcium while still preserving the crystalline scaffold

The initial carious lesion in dentin afflicts the tubuli that serve as a highway for bacteria to spread into the dentin. As the tubules of the carious dentin become more distended due to breakdown of their walls by the proteolytic enzymes excreted by the invading bacteria, they may fuse and form spindle-shaped cavities perpendicular to the tubules. Fusion of afflicted tubules over a longer distance may also create spindle-shaped cavities in the same direction as the tubuli run. Through the continued loss of dentin between the tubules, its inner structure crumbles away (Figs. 5.2a–d). When caries is not halted by dental treatment, bacteria and their toxic products will reach the soft inner part of the tooth, the dental pulp, and evoke an inflammatory response (pulpitis to be discussed later on, see Sect. 7.3). Subsequently, the pulp dies and toxic substances from the pulp space diffuse through the apical foramen into the adjacent periapical part of the periodontal ligament and surrounding jaw bone. Periapical disease will now ensue. If the root surface of a tooth is exposed due to periodontal disease (see Chap. 8), the root-covering caries may also be the victim of carious decay. At this site, the bacteria penetrate into the cementum using the collagen fibres that once anchored the tooth in its tooth socket as pathways.

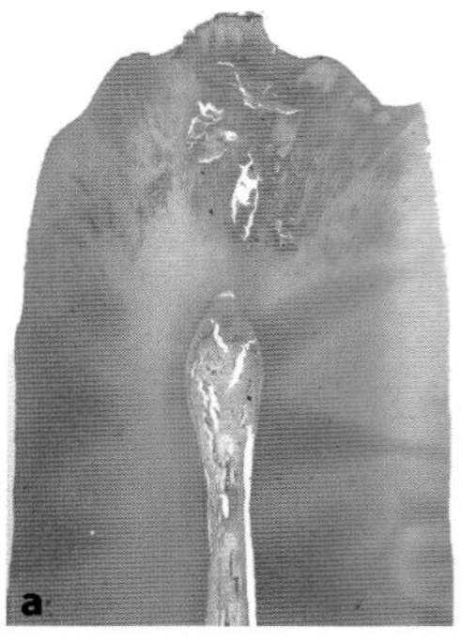

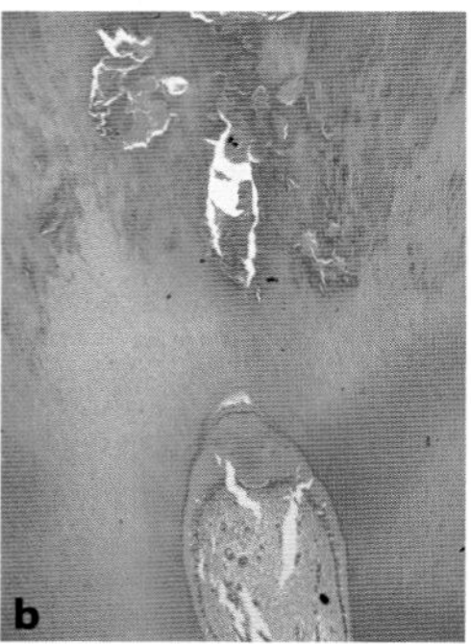

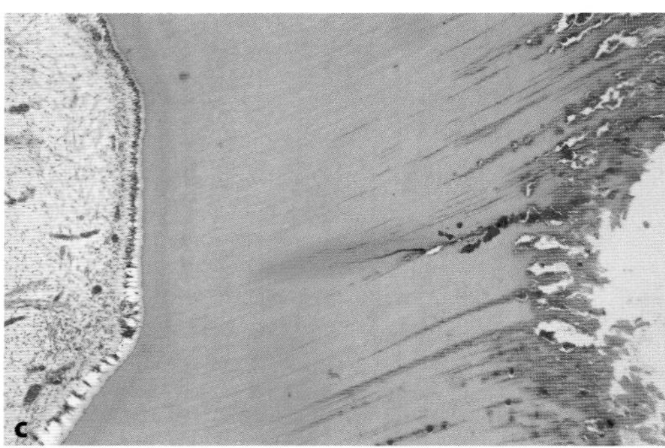

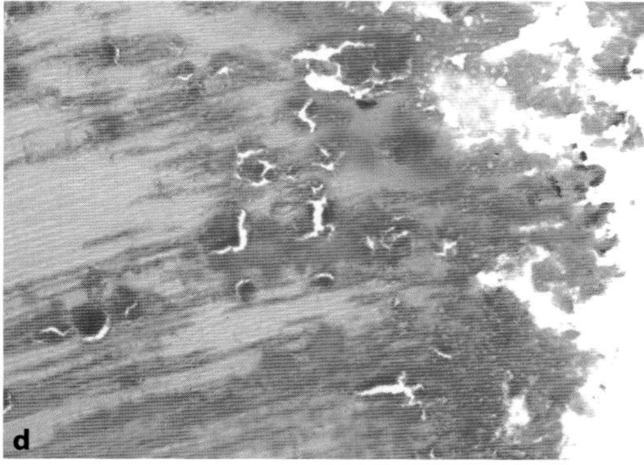

Fig. 5.2a–d Caries-induced alterations in dentin and dental pulp. **a** Low power view showing area of discoloration and disintegration. **b** Higher magnification showing also deposition of reparative dentin in the dental pulp. **c** Area of disintegration and dentin tubuli filled with bacteria extending towards the dental pulp. **d** In more advanced disintegration, transverse splits connect the widened tubuli

5.2 Attrition

Attrition is the gradual loss of dental hard tissue as a result of chewing [5]. Therefore, it only affects the tooth surfaces used in or shearing against each other during mastication: incisal for incisors and cuspids, occlusal for premolars and molars, and approximal (surfaces where adjacent teeth touch each other). When the enamel cap is worn away, the underlying dentin becomes exposed. Usually this shows a dark-brown discoloration (Fig. 5.3). The dental pulp compensates for the loss of dental hard tissues by the deposition of secondary dentin.

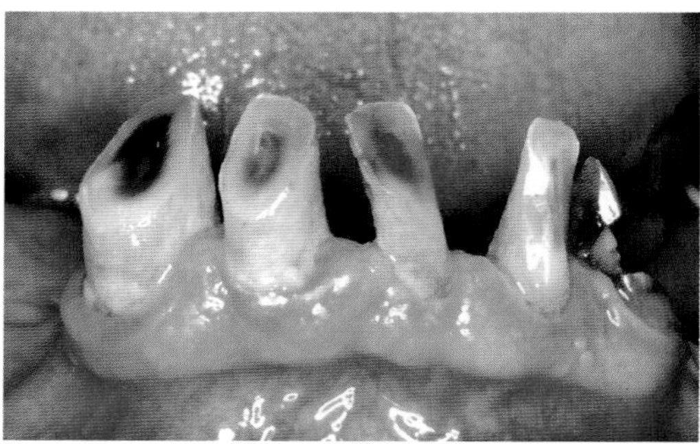

Fig. 5.3 Attrition: mandibular incisor teeth with enamel worn away thus exposing the brown discolored dentin

5.3 Abrasion

Abrasion is due to wearing away of dental hard tissue by causes other than mastication [5]. It may be due to improper use of the dentition such as holding items between the teeth such as pipes, hairpins, or other objects. The most common cause of abrasion is too vigorous toothbrushing that may cause defects at the necks of the teeth.

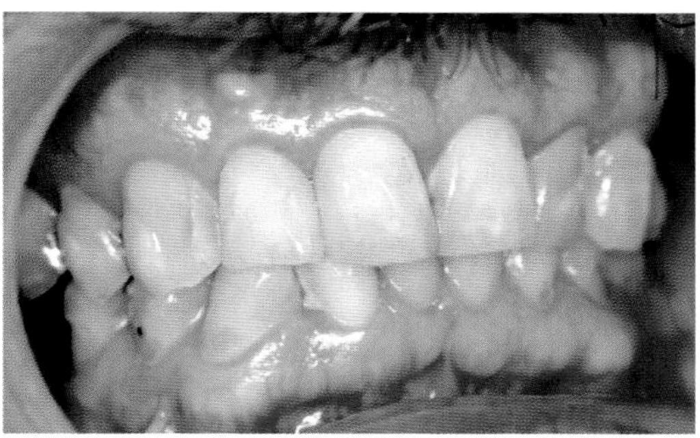

Fig. 5.4 Erosion: buccal surfaces of right maxillary cuspid and first premolar tooth showing loss of enamel. Both central and right lateral incisor teeth show white areas at their labial surfaces indicating incipient decalcification but still maintaining their crystalline structure

5.4 Erosion

Dental erosion is defined as loss of dental hard tissues due to chemical injuries other than those occurring in tooth caries [5]. Excessive intake of acid beverages or gastric reflux may cause this type of tooth damage as any solution of low pH may dissolve the enamel. In contrast to caries, which causes subsurface demineralisation, erosion is a surface phenomenon. The affected teeth show smoothly outlined defects that may involve not only enamel but also the underlying dentin at areas where the enamel has disappeared (Fig. 5.4).

5.5 Hypercementosis

During the lifetime of the teeth, continuous apposition of cementum on the root surface causes a gradual increase of its thickness. This gradual increase in cementum may compensate for loss of tooth tissue at the occlusal surface due to physiological tooth wear, thus maintaining the length of the tooth. Sometimes, this apposition of cementum is excessive, leading to a very thick cementum layer. This condition is termed hypercementosis (Fig. 5.5). This cementum usually is of the acellular type although sometimes cellular cementum resembling bone may also occur. Hypercementosis may occur without any recognisable cause, but it can also be seen with chronic periapical inflammation. Moreover, it occurs in patients with Paget's disease [7].

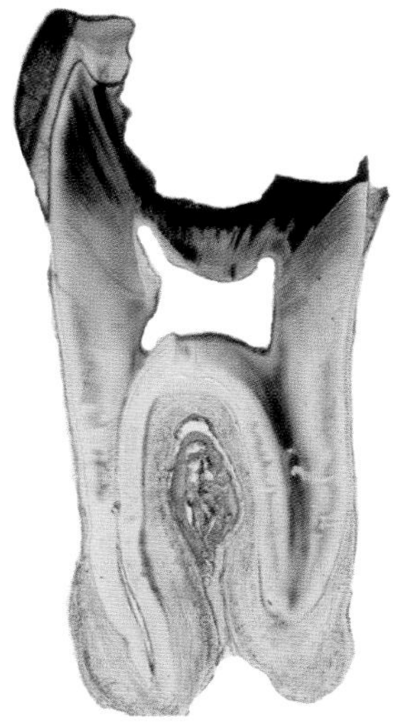

Fig. 5.5 Ground section showing molar tooth with carious decay and pronounced hypercementosis. Both roots are covered with a thick cementum layer, most pronounced in the apical area

5.6 Cementicles

Within the periodontal membrane, small, spherical calcified basophilic bodies may be seen. They may occur lying freely within the fibres of the periodontal ligament but can also be observed within the root-covering cementum layer or the bone of the alveolar socket (Figs. 5.6a, b).

5.7 Secondary and Tertiary Dentin Formation

As already briefly alluded to in Chap. 2, the bulk of the dentin is formed prior to tooth eruption. This is called primary dentin. Secondary dentin is the dentin that is formed during the lifetime

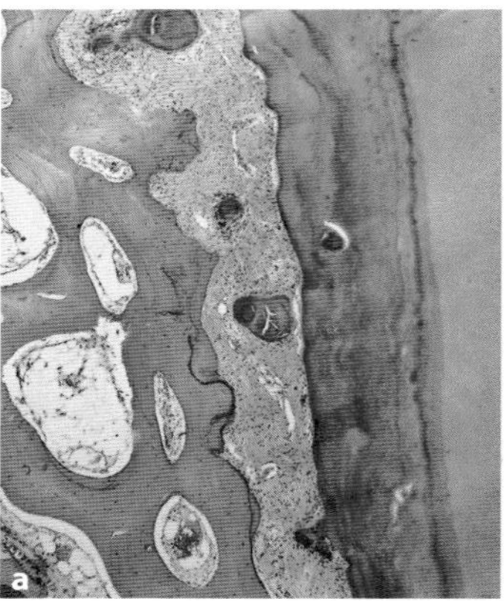

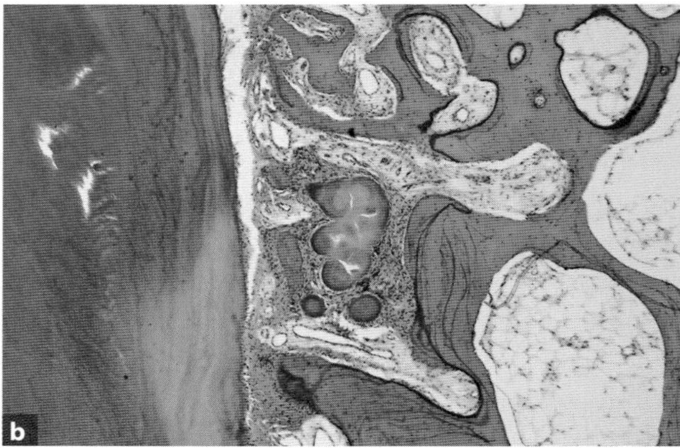

Fig. 5.6a,b Periodontal ligament space showing presence of spherical basophilic structures representing cementum deposits, the so-called cementicles. They may lie embedded in the collagenous fibres of the periodontal ligament or attached to or engulfed by the root cementum (**a**) but they can also be found more remote from the root surface surrounded by cancellous bone (**b**)

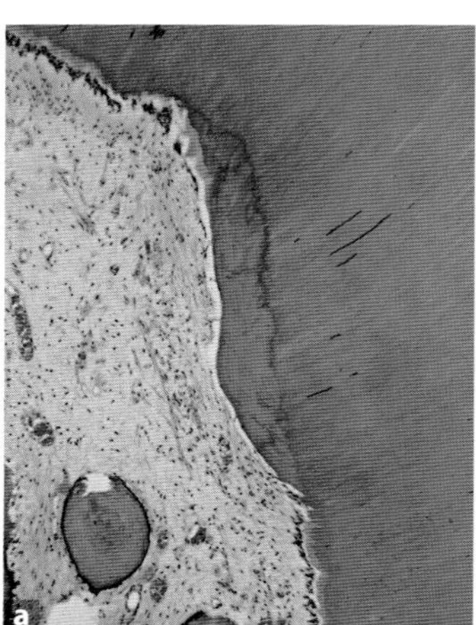

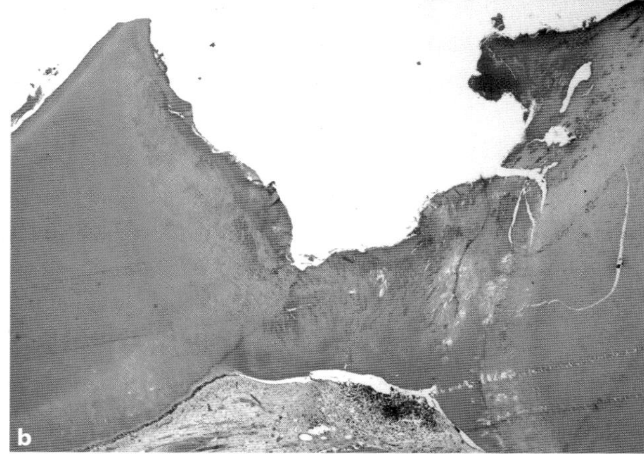

Fig. 5.7a,b Tertiary dentin showing absence of dentin tubuli. Also the odontoblastic rim is missing in this area (**a**). Sometimes, excessive deposition of tertiary dentin may wall of the dental pulp temporarily against the advancing carious decay (**b**)

of the teeth, possibly due to the minor mechanical and thermal injuries involved with tooth functioning. Its amount increases with age. As it occurs on each wall of the dental pulp, it causes gradual decrease of the size of the pulp chamber as well as the root canal. Secondary dentin contains less tubuli than primary dentin and a basophilic demarcation line similar to the reversal lines seen in bone usually separates the primary from the secondary dentin.

Tertiary dentin is formed in response to heavy pulp irritation, mostly occurring after loss of the protecting enamel cap. It only occurs at the site where the odontoblasts are injured. In tertiary dentin, the dental tubuli are greatly diminished in number and do not show the regular course from dental pulp to dentino-enamel junction. Sometimes, it may even contain cellular inclusions (Figs. 5.7a, b). Its formation may be considered a response of the pulp to injury aimed at protecting itself. It may also occur in response to the dentist's drilling and filling.

5.8 External Resorption

The dental hard tissues may be resorbed from their outside, in which case one speaks of external resorption. This is a physiological event responsible for the shedding of the deciduous teeth (Fig. 5.8) but when occurring in association with the permanent dentition, it may cause premature loss of the involved teeth. When the resorption takes place at the walls of the dental pulp chamber, the condition is called internal resorption. For discussion of this latter condition, see Chap. 7 on pulpal diseases. External resorption may occur at the surface of teeth buried in the jaw which have not erupted. It may also occur at the surface of erupted teeth, often as a late event after trauma, reimplantation after traumatic evulsion, root fracture, local inflammation, or due to a slowly expanding intraosseous jaw neoplasm. When no etiologic factor can be identified, the condition is called idiopathic. External idiopathic root resorption can further be defined according to the site affected as cervical, apical, or interradicular [1–4, 6].

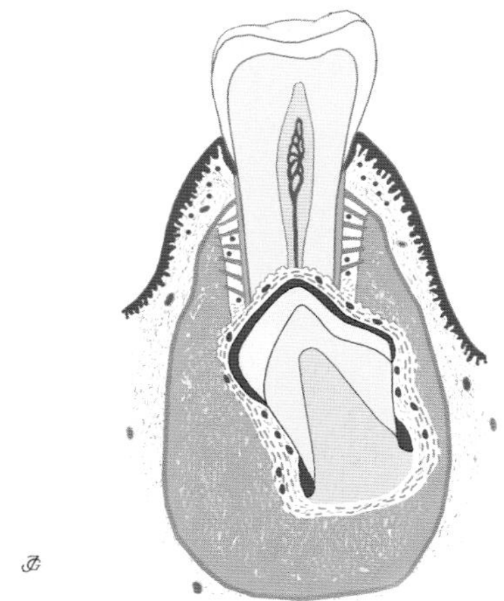

Fig. 5.8 External root resorption of deciduous teeth by underlying permanent successor. (Modified from drawing by John A.M. de Groot)

In invasive cervical resorption there is progressive loss of cementum and dentin in the cervical tooth region with replacement by fibrovascular tissue derived from the periodontal ligament, together with deposition of cementum-like hard tissue that may be mistaken for a fibro-osseous lesion (Figs. 5.9a–c) [2].

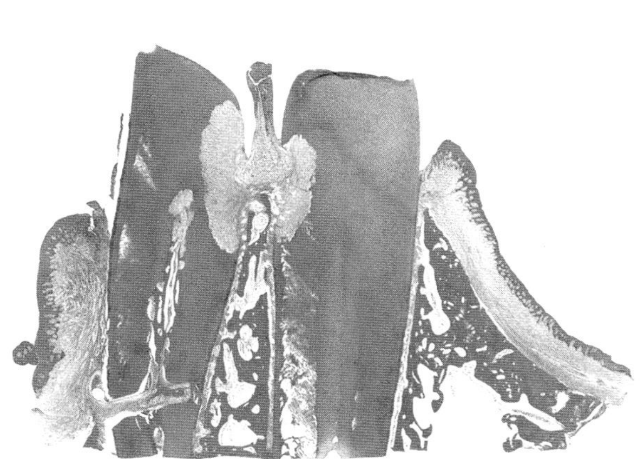

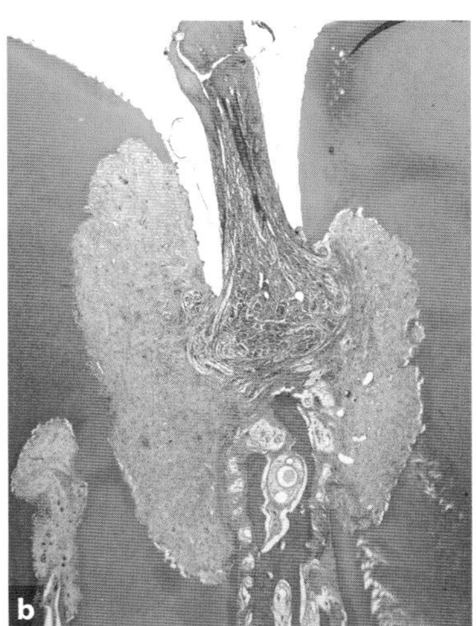

Fig. 5.9a–c Photomicrograph shows two neighbouring teeth separated by interdental gingiva and bony septum. Both teeth show cervical external resorption leading to surface defects filled with fibrous tissue. **a** Low power view, **b** Intermediate magnification, **c** *see next page*

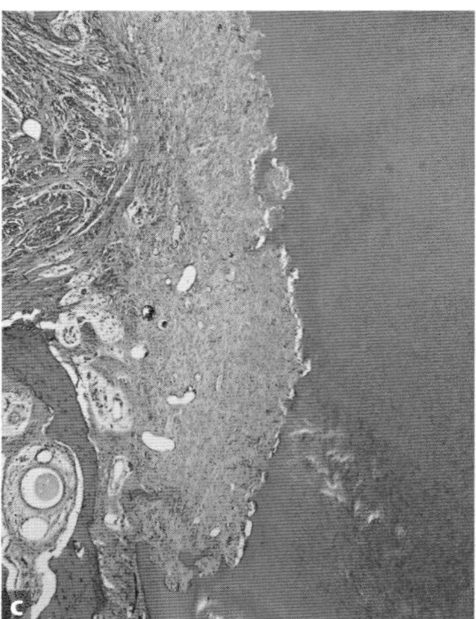

Fig. 5.9 *(continued)* Photomicrograph shows two neighbouring teeth separated by interdental gingiva and bony septum. Both teeth show cervical external resorption leading to surface defects filled with fibrous tissue. **c** Detail

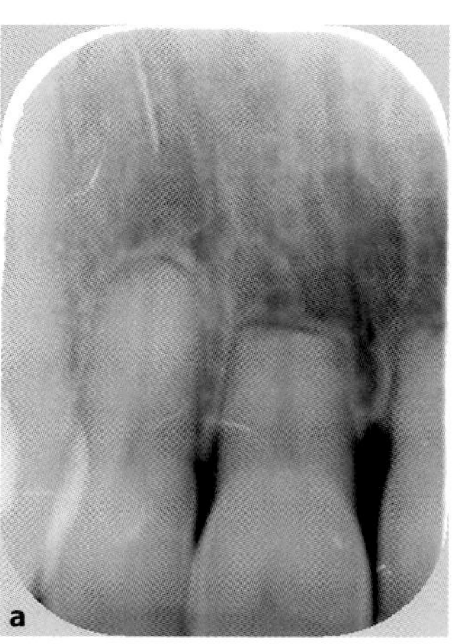

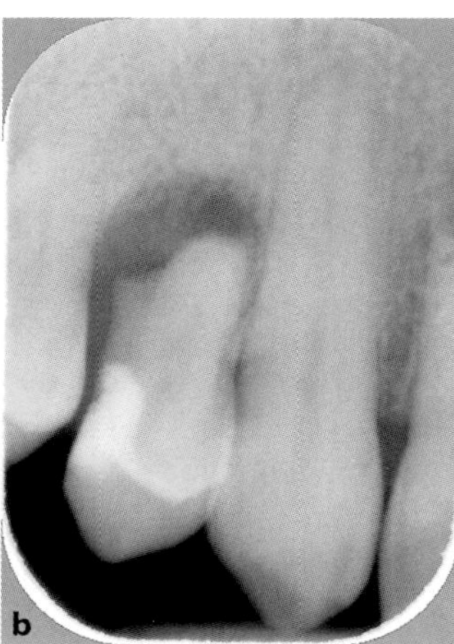

Fig. 5.10a,b Dental radiographs showing apical resorption: **a** Maxillary incisor teeth, **b** Maxillary first premolar tooth

In all cases of external resorption, the tooth is resorbed from the outside by osteoclastic (in fact odontoclastic) cells located in the periodontal ligament that at first attack the root cementum and thereafter the root dentin. It may cause complete loss of the entire dentition (Figs. 5.10a, b).

When examining teeth histologically, minute areas of root resorption subsequently repaired by cementum deposition can often be found (Fig. 5.11). These findings are not considered to represent examples of external resorption. To qualify for this diagnosis, gross defects in the root surface should be visible either at extracted teeth or at dental radiographs.

5.9 Tooth Fracture

Mechanical trauma may lead to fracture of the tooth. Fractures above the level of the gingival margin involve the tooth crown. Through the fracture line, bacteria may easily gain access to the inner part of the tooth and caries with consequent pulpitis may ensue, thus jeopardizing the vitality of the tooth pulp. In case of root fractures, the fixation of the tooth in its socket may serve as a splint. The fracture may heal by fibrous union or by the deposition of a dentin-like material (Figs. 5.12a, b).

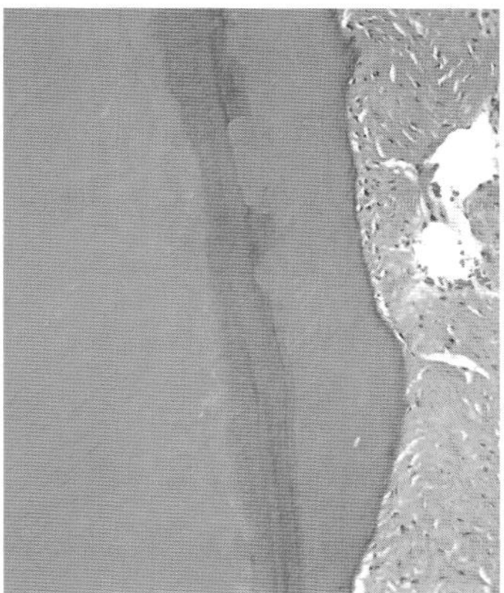

Fig. 5.11 Photomicrograph showing minute areas of resorption in the cementum layer adjacent to the dentin (lamellated basophilic) subsequently repaired by a covering of more eosinophilic cementum

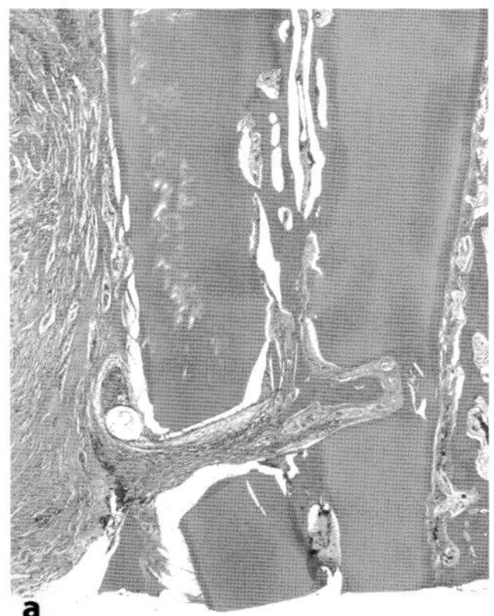

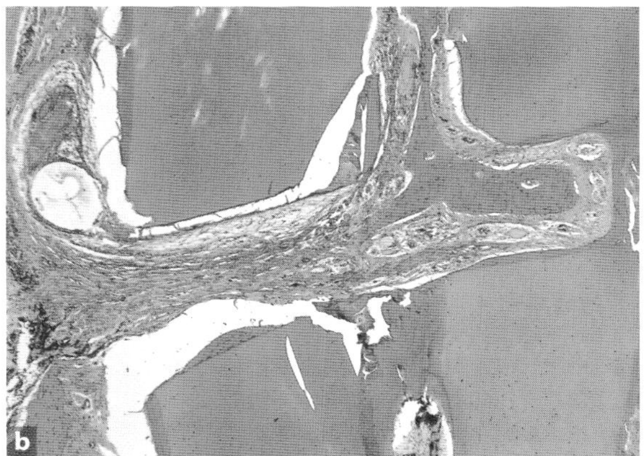

Fig. 5.12a,b Tooth fracture healed by fibrous union. **a** Overview showing fibrous tissue between upper and lower root part. **b** Detail displaying walling off of apical pulp part by tertiary dentin and bone formation in the upper part of the pulp and in the fibrous tissue bridging the gap between both root fragments. In the adjacent periodontal ligament, cystic degeneration of an epithelial rest of Malassez is visible

5.10 Pigmentations

Pigmentations of teeth may be due to the optical effect of disturbed enamel and/or dentin formation as is the case with dentinogenesis imperfecta, dentinal dysplasia, or enamel hypocalcification. It may also be due to the uptake of colored substances in defective enamel as is the case in amelogenesis imperfecta. Illustrations of these types of discoloration can be found in Chap. 4. It may also occur through coloring agents taken up by tooth formation [8–10]. From this latter group, tetracyclin is a prominent member and this topic will be discussed more extensively.

5.10.1 Tetracyclin Discoloration

Through binding to calcium, tetracyclin is deposited together with calcium in any tissue undergoing mineralisation. After its incorporation during mineralisation, it can be demonstrated in teeth and bones in ultraviolet light, showing up as fluorescent yellow bands. Grossly, tetracyclin causes a greyish-black discoloration of the tooth

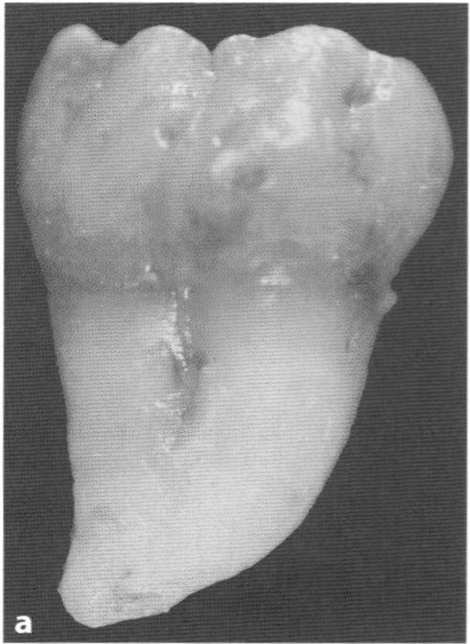

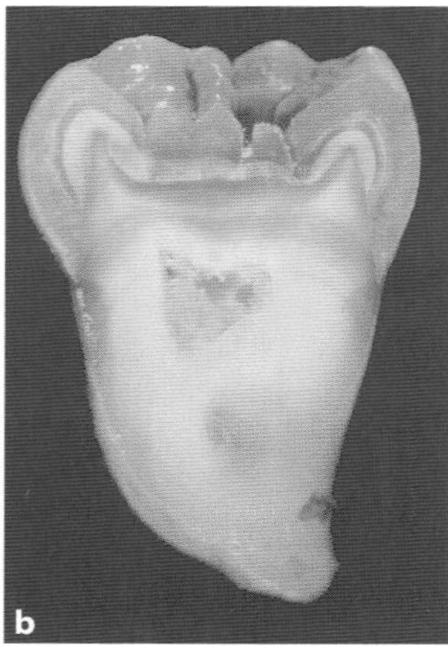

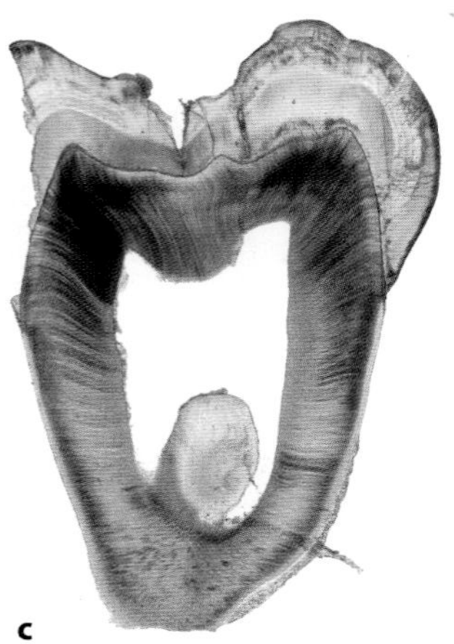

Fig. 5.13a–c Tetracyclin discoloration; **a** Outer view showing grey discoloration of crown and yellow discoloration of upper part of the root. **b** Cut surface showing the band-like appearance of the discoloration indicating several administrations of the drug. **c** Ground section also illustrating the band-like discolorations in the enamel and a tiny yellow line in the dentin

crown (Figs. 5.13a–c). When making ground sections of these teeth, the tetracyclin bands can be observed under UV light illumination both in dentin as well as in enamel, each band indicating a time point of tetracyclin administration. After decalcification the tetracyclin has been lost together with the calcium and therefore, in decalcified paraffin sections, this fluorescence is not present anymore.

References

1. Cholia SS, Wilson PHR, Makdissi J (2005) Multilple idiopathic external apical root resorption: report of four cases. Dentomaxillofac Radiol 34:240–246
2. Coyle M, Toner M, Barry H (2006) Multiple teeth showing invasive cervical resorption—an entity with little known histologic features. J Oral Pathol Med 35:55–57
3. Hartsfield JK, Everett ET, Al-Qawasami RA (2004) Genetic factors in external apical root resorption and orthodontic treatment. Crit Rev Oral Biol Med 15:115–122
4. Kerr DA, Courtney RM, Burkes EJ (1970) Multiple idiopathic root resorption. Oral Surg Oral Med Oral Pathol 29:552–565
5. Litonjua LA, Adnreana S, Bush PJ et al. (2003) Tooth wear: attrition, erosion, and abrasion. Quint Int 34:435–446
6. Ne RF, Witherspoon DE, Gutmann JL (1999) Tooth resorption. Quint Int 30:9–25
7. Rao VM, Karasick D (1982) Hypercementosis—An important clue to Paget disease of the maxilla. Skeletal Radiol 9:126–128
8. Sulieman M (2005) An overview of tooth discoloration. Extrinsic, intrinsic and internalized stains. Dental Update 32:463–471
9. Tahmassebi JF, Day PF, Toumba KJ et al. (2003) Paediatric dentistry in the new millennium: 6. Dental anomalies in children. Dental Update 30:534–540
10. Tredwin CJ, Scully C, Bagan-Sebastian JV (2005) Drug-induced disorders of teeth. J Dent Res 84:596–602

Chapter 6

Disturbed Tooth Eruption

6

Tooth eruption comprises the movement of teeth through the soft tissues of the jaw and the overlying mucosa into the oral cavity (Fig. 6.1) [1]. The involved biological processes are not yet entirely elucidated, but the importance of the dental follicle has been established beyond doubt. Teeth may erupt too early, too late, not in the proper position, or not at all. In the latter event, one speaks of impaction. This is most often seen in lower 3rd molar teeth.

6.1 Ankylosis

Ankylosis represents fusion of either enamel, dentin, or root cementum with adjacent alveolar bone (Figs. 6.2a–c). It may occur in impacted as well as in normally erupted teeth. It may be the result of any condition in which the vitality of the normally present intervening periodontal ligament has been jeopardized. Sometimes, ankylosis occurs in combination with external resorption. The role of the epithelial rests of Malassez in preventing ankylosis has already been mentioned before (see Chap. 1).

6.2 Premature Eruption

Both deciduous as well as permanent teeth may erupt into the oral cavity at a too-early age. Because the roots are not yet well developed at that time, the fixation of the tooth in the jaw may be compromised and the subsequent root development may be disturbed, resulting in teeth with malformed and/or too-short roots.

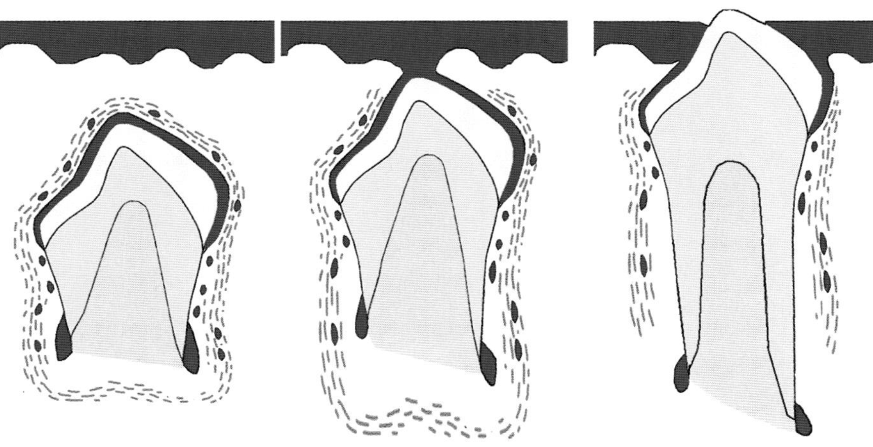

Fig. 6.1 Schematic drawing showing movement of tooth germ through oral epithelium during successive stages of eruption

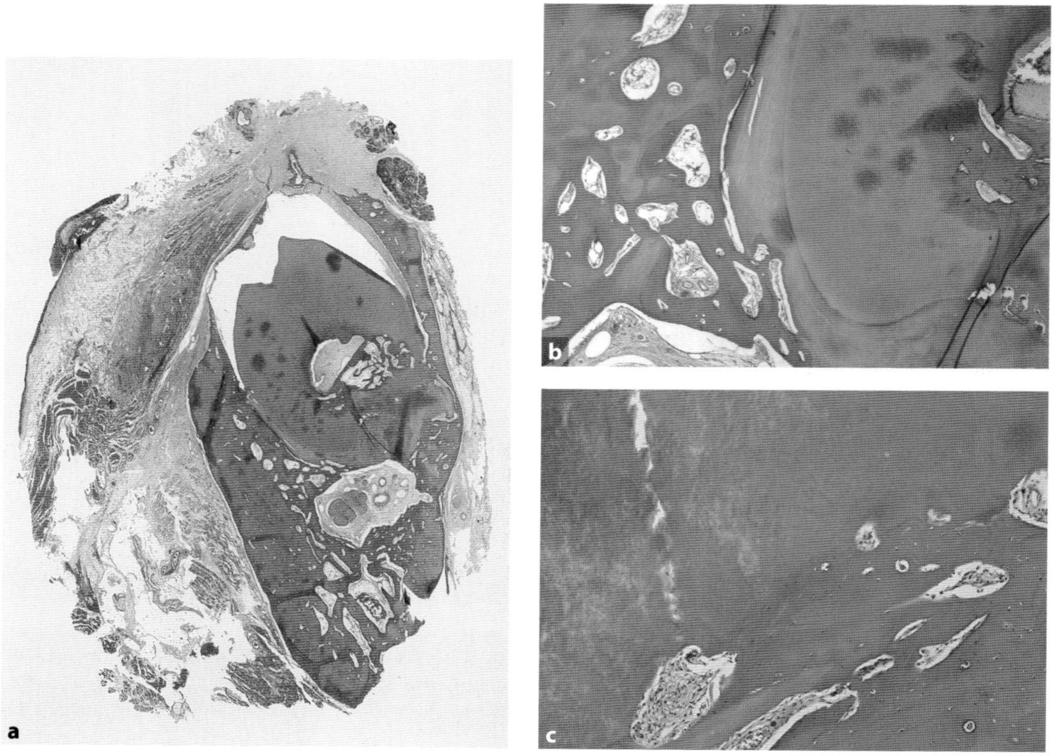

Fig. 6.2 Continuity between root surface covering cementum and bone of the alveolar socket displayed in low (**a**), intermediate (**b**), and higher power (**c**) view

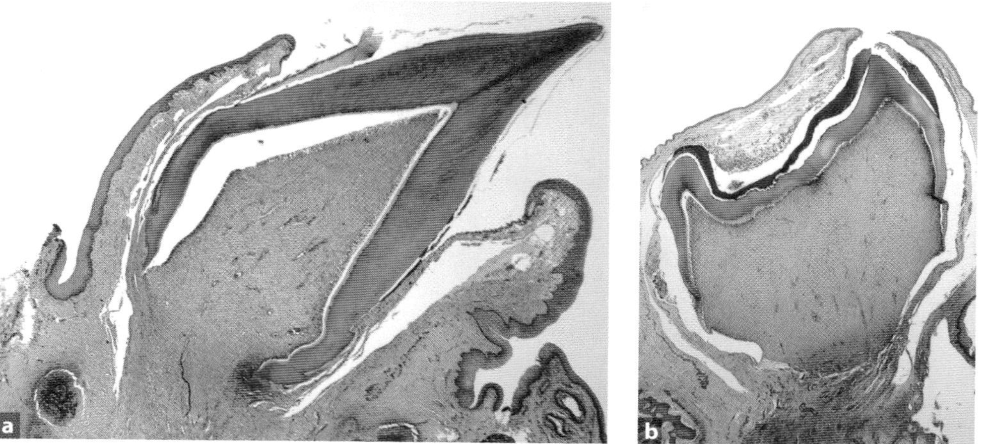

Fig. 6.3a,b Premature eruption of teeth in Hallermann Streiff syndrome. **a** Incisor tooth piercing through the oral mucosa. **b** Molar tooth still covered by soft tissues for the major part. Both teeth lack a properly formed rooth, only connected to the jaw bone by a fibrous stalk

Sometimes, the teeth exfoliate spontaneously due to lack of a well-formed root and periodontal ligament. Premature eruption may occur as one of the abnormalities of the Hallermann-Streiff syndrome (Figs. 6.3a, b) [2].

Within the differential diagnosis of spontaneously exfoliating teeth, one should discern between loss of tooth fixation due to external resorption or to root maldevelopment. In the former case, histologic examination shows an irregular outer tooth surface with Hownship's lacunae while in the latter, poorly deformed dentin containing cellular inclusions may be found. Root maldevelopment not only occurs in case of premature eruption but also in various forms of inherited disorders of dentin formation already mentioned (see Sect. 4.2).

6.3 Local Conditions Causing Disturbed Eruption

Teeth may erupt at the wrong place or not at all if local conditions interfere with the eruption pathway. Usually, these are diseases of the jaw bone or the overlying soft tissues. Also, odontogenic tumours arising around the crown area of a developing teeth may hinder proper eruption. Quite often, the failure of a tooth to erupt will be the first sign of such a jaw tumour.

Eruption of a tooth in an aberrant position more often is due to jaw lesions lying adjacent to the developing roots than to obstacles in the eruption pathway. Description of the various jaw conditions that may interfere with tooth eruption can be found in textbooks on oral or head and neck pathology.

References

1. Craddock HL, Youngson CC (2004) Eruptive tooth movement—the current state of knowledge. Br Dent J 197:385–391
2. Slootweg PJ, Huber J (1984) Dento-alveolar abnormalities in oculomandibulodyscephaly (Hallermann-Streiff Syndrome). J Oral Pathol 13:147–154

Chapter 7

Disorders of the Dental Pulp

7

Pulpal diseases may be either inflammatory or degenerative. Very rarely, jaw tumours may grow through the apical foramen into the pulp space (Figs. 7.1a, b).

7.1 Pulp Stones, False and True (Denticles)

Denticles are calcified masses in the dental pulp. One discerns between true denticles that have tubules like dentin and false denticles that have a concentrically lamellated structure. Irrespective of being identifiable as true or false, they may lie free in the dental pulp, being connected with the wall of the pulp chamber, or lie entirely within the dentin in case of formation of excessive secondary or tertiary dentin. Depending on this topographical relationship with the tooth, they are classified as either free, attached, or embedded (Figs. 7.2a, b).

In addition to calcifications in the form of denticles, the pulp may contain diffuse calcifications, occurring as metaplastic ossification along collagen fibres or blood vessels. Through merging of these calcifications with each other, large masses may form (Fig. 7.3). However, they lack the inner structure and circumscribed nature shown by the true or false denticles.

7.2 Internal Resorption

In case of internal resorption, the dental pulp transforms into granulation tissue with multinucleated osteoclasts accumulating at the pulpo-dentinal border. There, they resorb the dentin, thus increasing the size of the pulp chamber [1]. Simultaneously, irregular masses of hard tissue resembling both bone and dentin may be formed haphazardly in the enlarged pulp chamber, partly onto the pulp wall, but also

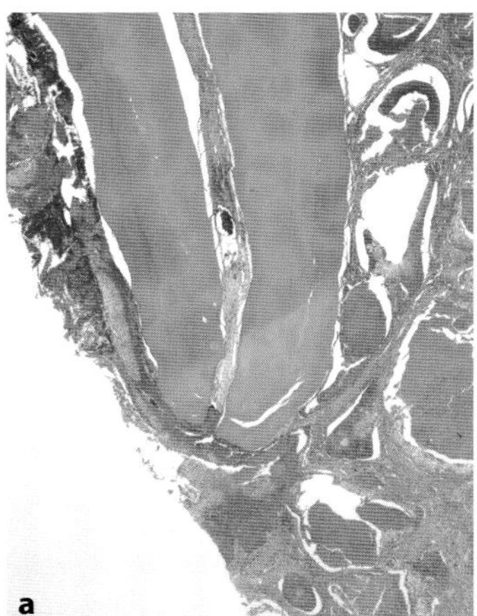

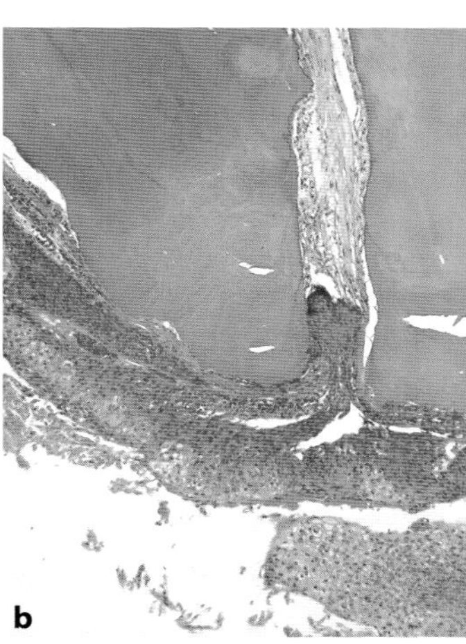

Fig. 7.1 Squamous cell carcinoma invading the tooth pulp through the apical foramen shown in low (**a**) and higher (**b**) magnification

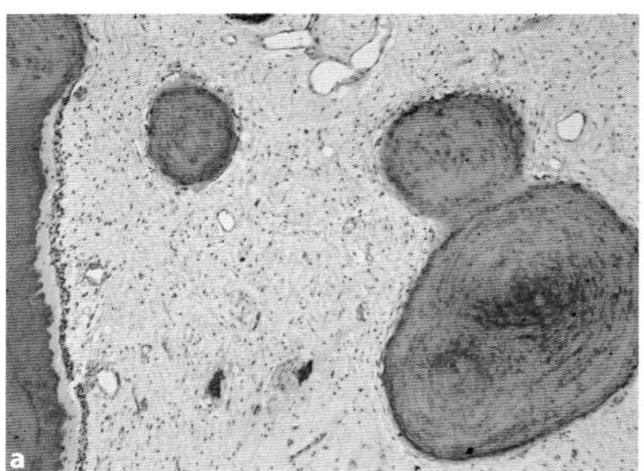

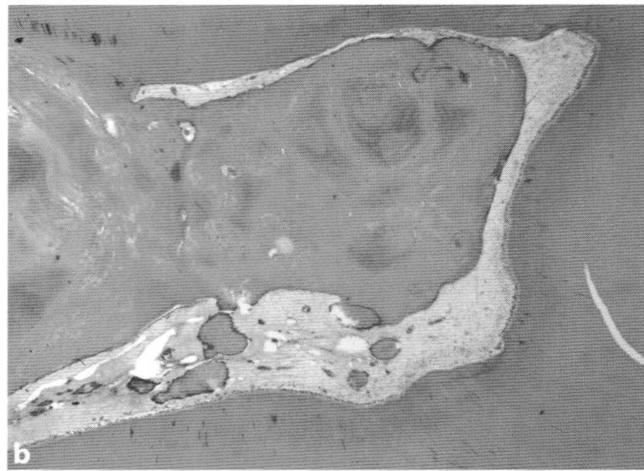

Fig. 7.2a,b The pulp may contain calcified aggregates representing poorly structured dentin. These denticles may lie free in the pulp (**a**) or attached to the pulp wall (**b**). In **b** is also shown that they may cause subtotal pulp obliteration. As these masses do not display regularly arranged dentin tubuli, they should be classified as false denticles

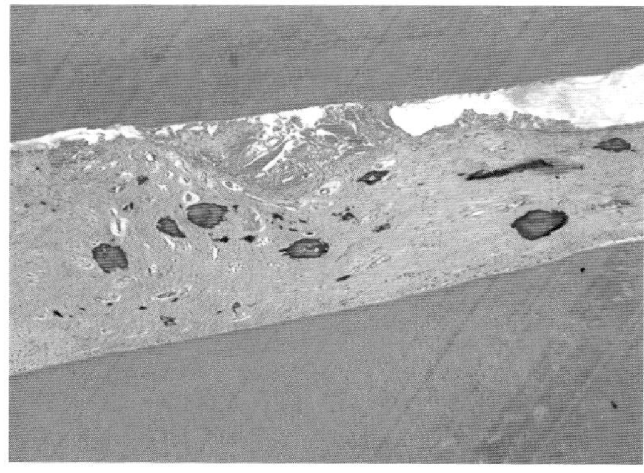

Fig. 7.3 The pulp may also contain amorphous calcified deposits. These are not real denticles

free (Figs. 7.4a–c). Functionally, this hard tissue deposition does not have any reparative properties. After resorption of a sufficient amount of dentin, the highly vascularised granulation tissue may be seen through the remaining translucent enamel as a pink spot.

Internal resorption may be seen as a sequel to dental trauma with intrapulpal hemorrhage. It may also result from chronic inflammation of the pulp.

7.3 Pulpitis

Mostly, pulpitis is due to caries, disappearance of the protective barrier of enamel and dentin allowing bacteria to reach the dental pulp. Rarely, it is due to thermal or mechanical trauma, either spontaneously occurring or due to dental treatment. Due to its distinctive anatomical position within the tooth, the chances of the pulp overcoming a bacterial infection are few. Oedema invariably connected with inflammation will compress capillaries and veins, thus compromising the blood supply of the pulp. Therefore, pulpitis usually results in pulp necrosis with periapical disease as an outcome. A brief description of this latter condition will follow in Sect. 7.3.1.

Histologically, pulpitis does not show any differences from inflammatory infiltrates found elsewhere in the body (Fig. 7.5). It may be classified as either acute, subacute, or chronic depending on the composition of the inflammatory infiltrate. Sometimes, abscess formation may occur. The odontoblasts that line the pulp chamber have usually disappeared. Areas of tertiary dentin may still be observed as a consequence of their past activities to wall off the pulp against the carious attack. Only in very mild inflammatory changes,

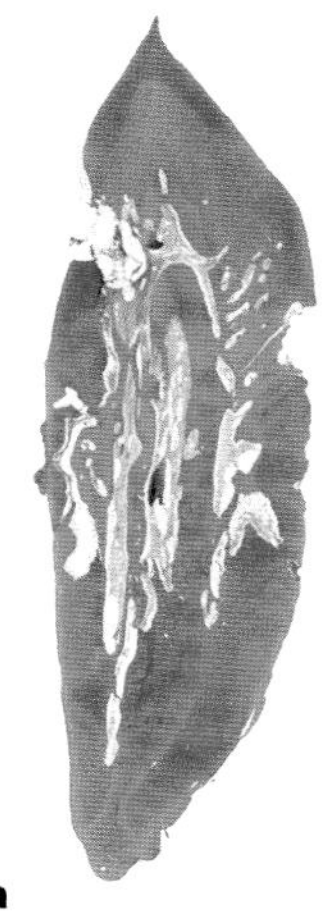

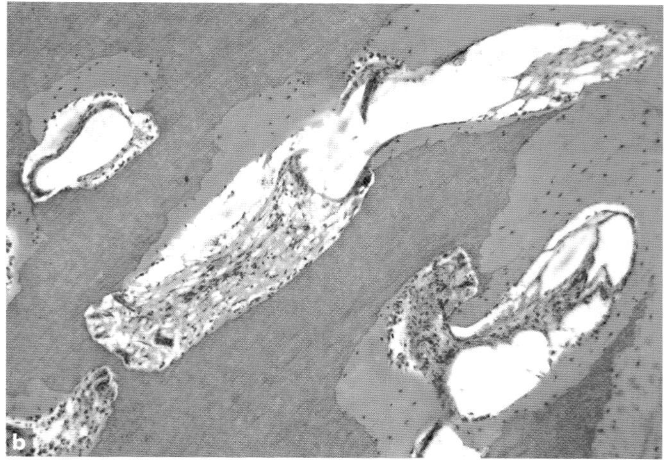

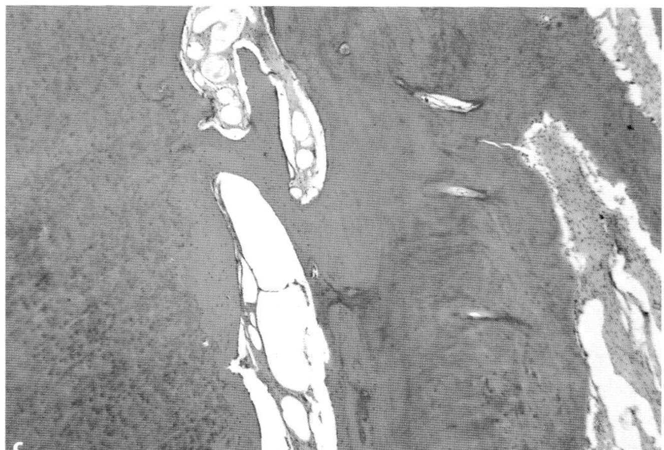

Fig. 7.4a–c In case of internal resorption the tooth is hollowed out by growth of fibrous tissue in which bone is deposited. **a** Overview, **b** Detail to show bone deposited onto remnants of dentin, **c** High power view to show the differences between tubular dentin and bone with cellular inclusions

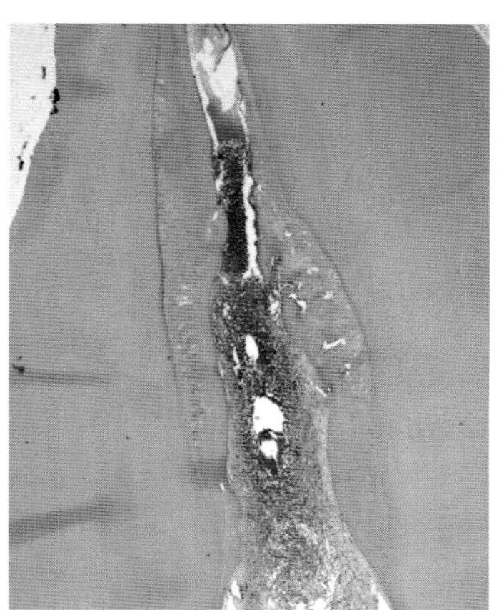

Fig. 7.5 Photomicrograph showing pulp tissue densely infiltrated by inflammatory cells. Pulp walls show covering with tertiary dentin

the odontoblastic layer lining the pulpal wall may be preserved, in that case, however, usually showing discontinuities and displacement of nuclei into the adjacent dentinal tubuli. Underlying capillaries may show some dilatation.

7.3.1 Periapical Disease

Triggered by bacteria or their toxic products that diffuse through the apical foramen, the periapical tissues respond by chronic inflammation and bone resorption. In this way, a cavity is formed lying adjacent (Figs. 7.6a, b) to the root tip and filled with granulation tissue, the so-called apical granuloma. Also, cell rests of Malassez lying in or in the vicinity of the periapical area may show reactive proliferation leading to the formation of a cystic cavity, the radicular cyst. When the noxious stimulus is removed by cleaning and filling the pulpal space, the inflammation may subside and complete healing can occur. Sometimes however, the granulation tissue is not replaced by new periapical bone but by fibrosis; in such instances a periapical scar is formed.

Usually, it is only the jaw bone that is resorbed in case of periapical disease, the root of the tooth being more resistent. That does not mean that roots of the teeth are immune to resorption. This condition has already been described before (see Sect. 5.8).

7.4 Pulp Polyp

Usually, inflammation of the pulp results in pulp necrosis as inflammatory alterations with their inherent oedema lead to increased tissue pressure in the pulp chamber reducing its blood supply. Only in situations where pulp tissue is not enclosed by the walls of the pulp chamber at each side, may inflamed pulp tissue transform into granulation tissue that protrudes into the oral cavity. This can only occur when large areas of dentin are lost due to caries. Sometimes these pulpal polyps may be partly covered by squamous epithelium, possibly due to the settling of viable squamous cells that are scraped off from the adjacent buccal epithelium by the sharp edges of the tooth cavity from which the polyp protrudes (Figs. 7.7a, b).

References

1. Ne RF, Witherspoon DE, Gutmann JL (1999) Tooth resorption. Quint Int 30:9–25

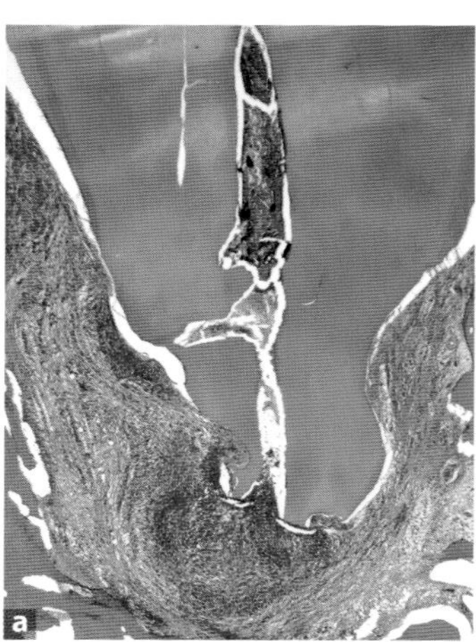

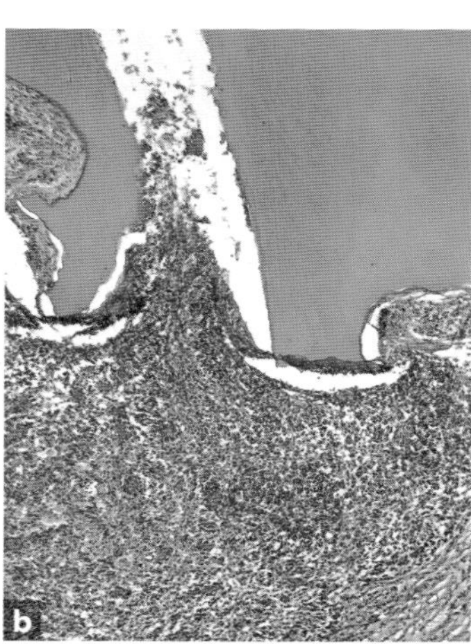

Fig. 7.6 Photomicrograph showing periapical granuloma (**a**). In higher magnification (**b**), slight external resorption of the root tip is shown

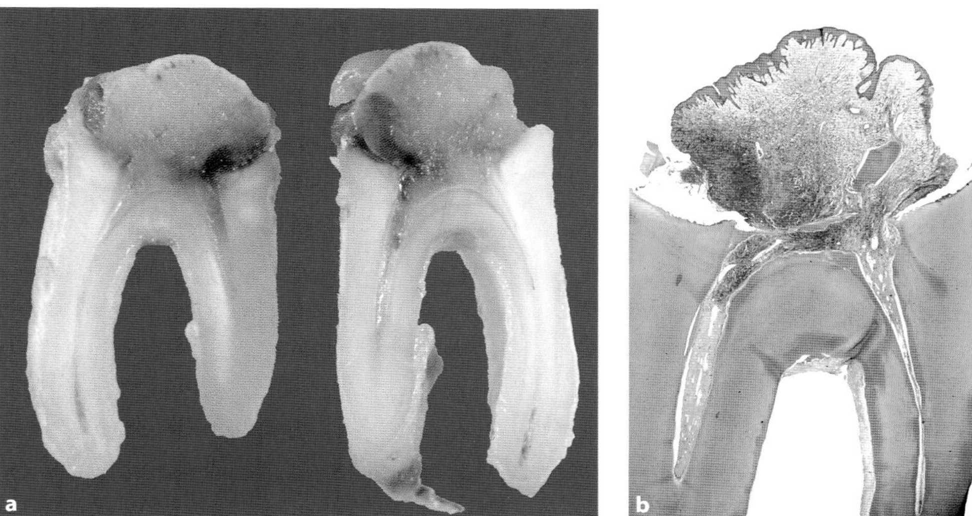

Fig. 7.7 **a** Cut surface showing soft tissue mass protruding from pulp cavity. **b** Histology shows granulation tissue covered with squamous epithelium

Chapter 8

Disorders of the Periodontal Tissues

8

Disorders of the periodontal tissues can be divided into diseases of the marginal gingiva proper and those also involving the underlying bone of the alveolar socket. Gingival diseases may be either hyperplastic or inflammatory. Periodontal disease is characterised by inflammation and breakdown of bone. Osseous dysplasia may be considered as a hamartoma of the periodontal tissues being composed of connective tissue, bone, and cementum. Many systemic disorders may impact the periodontal tissues [1]. Most of them do not result in histologic alterations that differ from the common inflammatory changes, excluding a few such as haematological malignancies, amyloidosis, and Ehlers-Danlos syndrome [2].

8.1 Gingival Inflammation

Gingival inflammation usually is caused by accumulation of bacterial plaque at the adjacent tooth surface. This plaque may be seen in histologic sections as a deep-blue mass lying at the surface of the tooth. Toxins of these bacteria as well as enzymes from the attracted neutrophils cause damage to the junctional epithelium that loses its fixation to the tooth. In this way, a niche is created between gingiva and tooth in which further plaque accumulation may occur. The thin layer of junctional epithelium becomes spongiotic and hyperplastic and may even disappear, resulting in ulceration. Also, elongated rete ridges develop that penetrate into the underlying fibrous tissue forming the bulk of the free gingiva. In this connective tissue, an inflammatory infiltrate evolves that may be either acute, subacute, or chronic (Figs. 8.1a, b). In due time, the inflammation involves the underlying periodontal bone that will be resorbed, thus causing loss of the fixation of the tooth in the jaw bone. At this stage, gingivitis has evolved into periodontitis, which is discussed in Sect. 8.3.

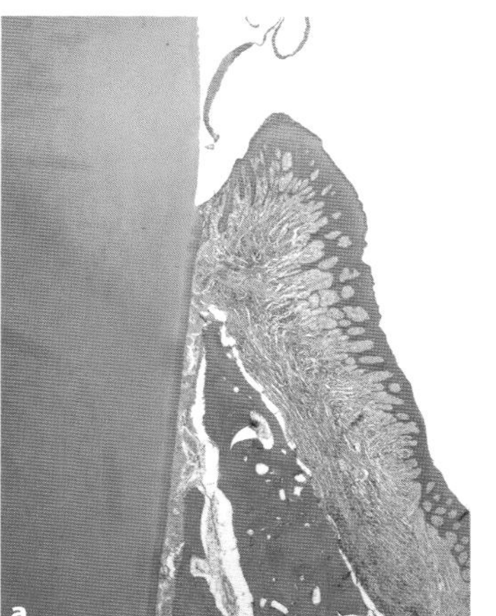

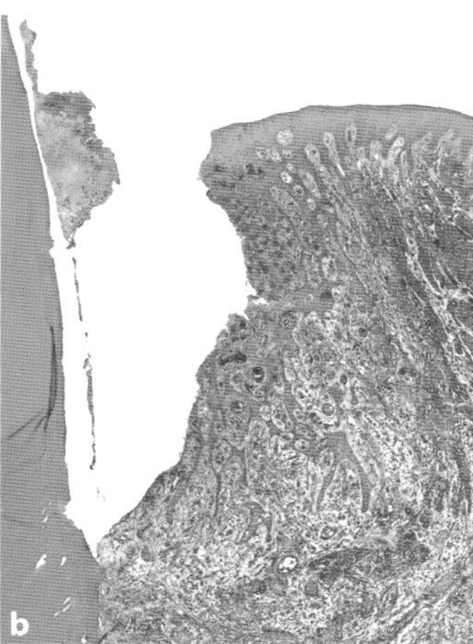

Fig. 8.1 Healthy gingival attachment (a) compared with gingival inflammation (**b**). In the normal situation, the junctional epithelium is only a thin cell layer with some rete ridges extending into the underlying gingival fibrous tissue. In case of gingivitis, the epithelium becomes spongiotic and hyperplastic and the underlying stroma is densely infiltrated with lymphocytes and plasmacells

8.2 Gingival Hyperplasia

Gingival hyperplasia may be generalised, in which case one speaks of gingival fibromatosis (Fig. 8.2). It may also occur confined to a limited area of the jaw; then it is called an epulis fibrosa (Fig. 8.3). In both cases, there is an increase in collagenous tissue with a varying cellularity. Due to the swelling of the gingival tissues, tooth cleaning is hampered. Consequently, bacterial plaque accumulates in the cleft between the tooth surface and the swollen gingival tissue. Therefore, the tissue facing the tooth surface usually shows reactive hyperplasia or even ulceration of the covering squamous epithelium, whereas the underlying stroma harbours an inflammatory infiltrate that may be either acute, subacute, or chronic. In fibrous epulides, the inflammatory alterations may sometimes be so extensive that the entire lesion is transformed into a lump of granulation tissue. In that case, the term epulis granulomatosa is used. Also, mineralised material resembling bone and cementum may be found in these fibrous epulides as well as nests and strands of odontogenic epithelium derived from the dental lamina.

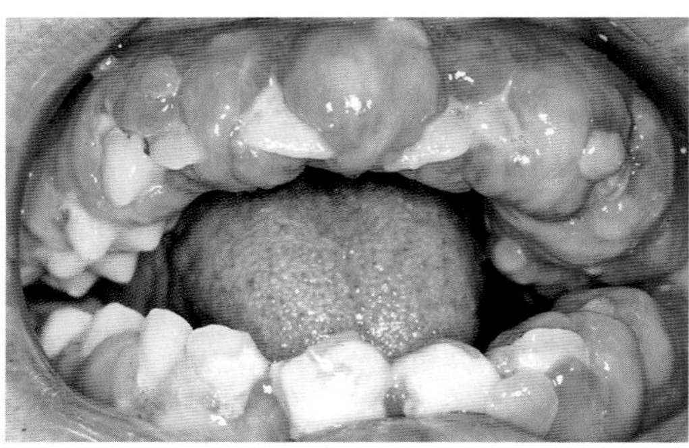

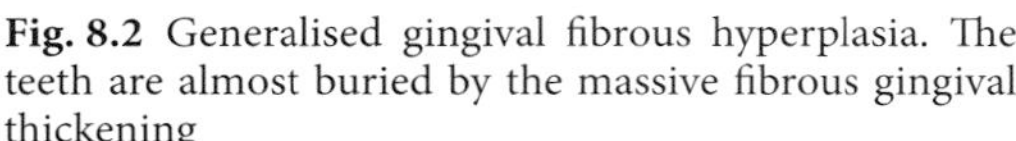

Fig. 8.2 Generalised gingival fibrous hyperplasia. The teeth are almost buried by the massive fibrous gingival thickening

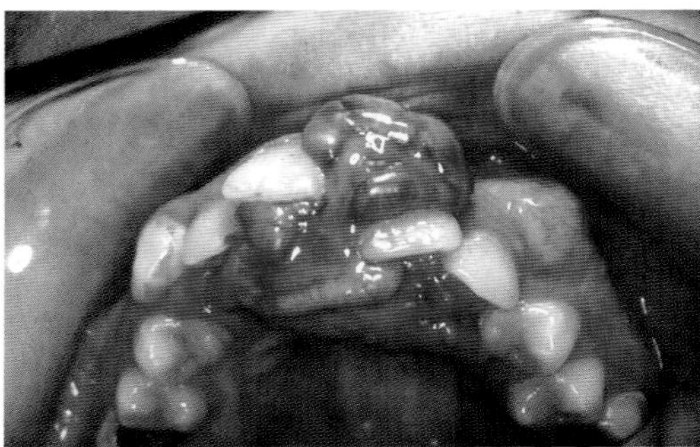

Fig. 8.3 Localised gingival fibrous hyperplasia. The lesion has caused displacement of the adjacent teeth

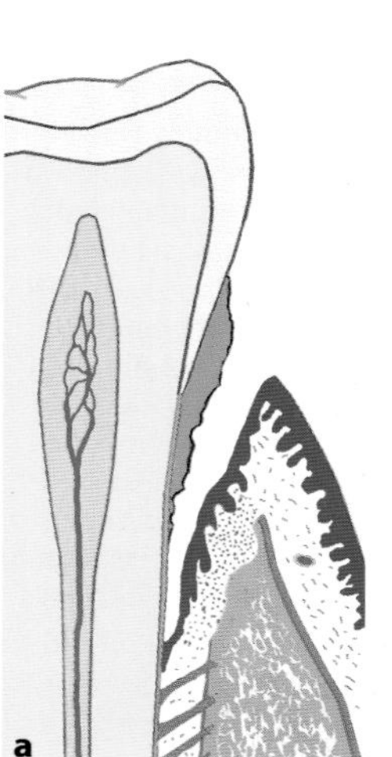

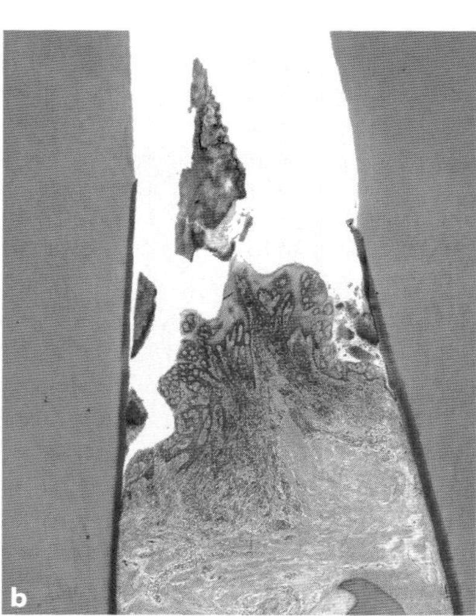

Fig. 8.4 a Detachment of gingiva from tooth surface and downward displacement of epithelial attachment (plaque accumulation in *green*). **b** Photomicrograph of interdental gingiva that has moved apically to leave the root cementum on both bordering teeth exposed to the oral cavity

8.3 Periodontitis

Periodontitis is the common sequel to chronic gingivitis and is recognised histologically by evidence of damage to the alveolar bone, associated with signs of chronic inflammation. The bone of the alveolar crest shows resorption as demonstrated by the presence of Hownship's lacunae sometimes still containing multinucleated osteoclasts. The epithelial attachment that normally lies in contact with the tooth enamel has moved downwards to be partly opposite the enamel and the root cementum or even entirely opposite the root cementum (Figs. 8.4a, b). Resorption of bone and downward displacement of the epithelial attachment may continue until there is insufficient periodontal tissue left for adequate fixation of the tooth in the jaw. Caries may add to the damage caused by periodontitis by attacking the cementum covering the exposed root surface.

8.4 Osseous Dysplasia

Osseous dysplasia represents a pathologic process of unknown etiology located in the tooth-bearing jaw areas in the immediate vicinity of the tooth apices and is thought to arise as the result of a proliferation of periodontal ligament fibroblasts that may deposit bone as well as cementum (Fig. 8.5). The condition occurs in various clinical forms that bear different names. However, all have the same histomorphology: cellular fibrous tissue, trabeculae of woven as well as lamellar bone, and spherules of cementum-like material. The ratio of fibrous tissue to mineralised material may vary and it has been shown that these lesions are initially fibroblastic, but over the course of several years may show increasing degrees of calcification. This variation in ratio of soft tissue to hard tissue is reflected in the radiographic appearance; lesions in the tooth-bearing jaw area may be either predominantly radiolucent, predominantly radiodense, or mixed.

Osseous dysplasia lacks encapsulation or demarcation but tends to merge with the adjacent cortical or medullary bone.

The several subtypes of osseous dysplasia are distinguished by clinical and radiological features. When occuring in the anterior mandible and involving only a few adjacent teeth, it is called *periapical osseous dysplasia.* A similar limited lesion occurring in a posterior jaw quadrant is known as *focal cemento-osseous dysplasia.* Lesions occuring bilaterally in the mandible or even involving all four jaw quadrants, are known as *florid osseous dysplasia* and *familial gigantiform cementoma.* The former is nonexpansile, involves two or more jaw quadrants, and occurs in middle-aged black females. The latter is expansile, involves multiple quadrants, and occurs at a young age. This type of osseous dysplasia shows an autosomal dominant inheritance with variable expression but sporadic cases without a history of familial involvement have also been reported. More extensive discussion of osseous dysplasia and its relationship with other bone-forming jaw lesions can be found in current textbooks on head and neck pathology [3].

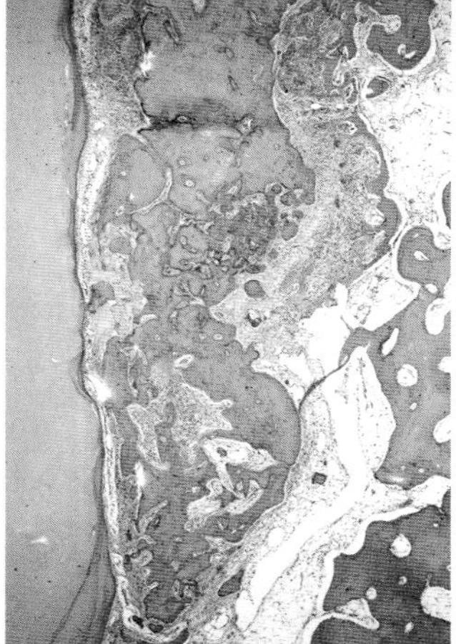

Fig. 8.5 Osseous dysplasia: hard tissue with histomorphology intermediate between bone and cementum interposed between root surface and jaw bone and causing widening of the periodontal ligament space

References

1. Jordan RC (2004) Diagnosis of periodontal manifestations of systemic diseases. Review. Periodontol 2000; 34:217–229
2. Slootweg PJ, Beemer FA (1986) Gingival fibrinoid deposits in Ehlers-Danlos Syndrome. J Oral Pathol 16:150–152
3. Slootweg PJ (2005) Osseous dysplasias. In: Barnes L, Eveson JW, Reichart P et al. (eds) World Health Organization Classification of Tumours. Pathology and Genetics of Head and Neck Tumours. IARC Press, Lyon. p 323

Chapter 9

Odontogenic Cysts

9

Cysts of the jaws are classified in several categories depending on histogenesis and etiology. Those that arise from odontogenic epithelium are called odontogenic; those that have their source in other epithelial structures are known as non-odontogenic [20]. The latter will not be discussed here. Within the odontogenic cysts, one discerns between developmental and inflammatory.

9.1 Odontogenic Cysts—Inflammatory

9.1.1 Radicular Cyst

Radicular cysts are located at the root tips of teeth in which the pulp has become necrotic, mostly due to advanced tooth caries (Figs. 9.1, 9.2). They arise from the epithelial rests of Malassez and develop when pulpal inflammation has led to to the formation of a periapical granuloma. Remnants of Hertwig's epithelial root sheath lying within this granuloma may proliferate due to the inflammatory stimulus and through subsequent liquefaction necrosis in the center of these enlarged epithelial nests, a fluid-filled cyst with an epithelial lining forms (Figs. 9.3a, b).

Radicular cysts are lined by nonkeratinising squamous epithelium. This epithelial lining may be thin and atrophic but, especially in case of inflammatory changes in the underlying connective tissue, the cyst epithelium shows proliferating rete processes that may form arcades. In many cysts, cholesterol clefts with adjacent giant cells occur. Within the cyst epithelium, hyaline bodies of various size and shape may be present (Figs. 9.4a–c).

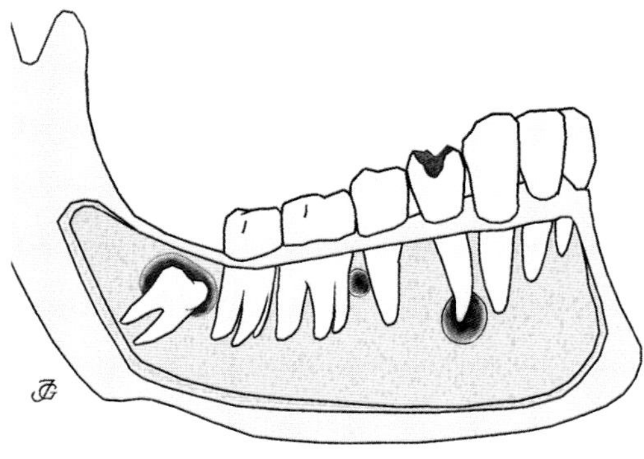

Fig. 9.1 Anatomical relationship between cysts and teeth. From *left* to *right*: dentigerous cyst surrounding crown of unerupted molar tooth, lateral periodontal cyst lying between roots of healthy teeth and radicular cyst at the root tip of a tooth with carious decay. (From [20] with permission)

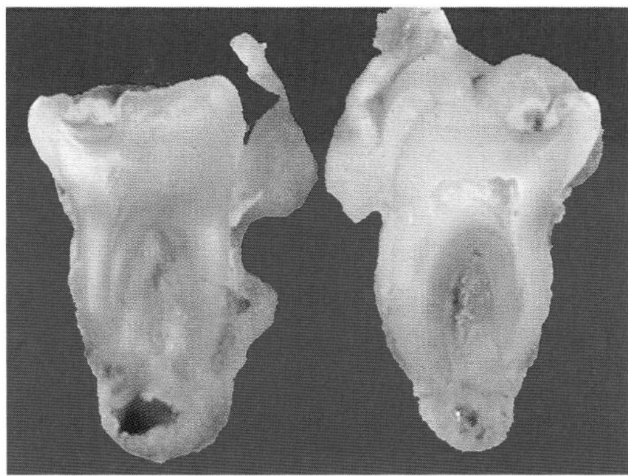

Fig. 9.2 Radicular cyst. Thick-walled cyst at the apex of a bisected tooth

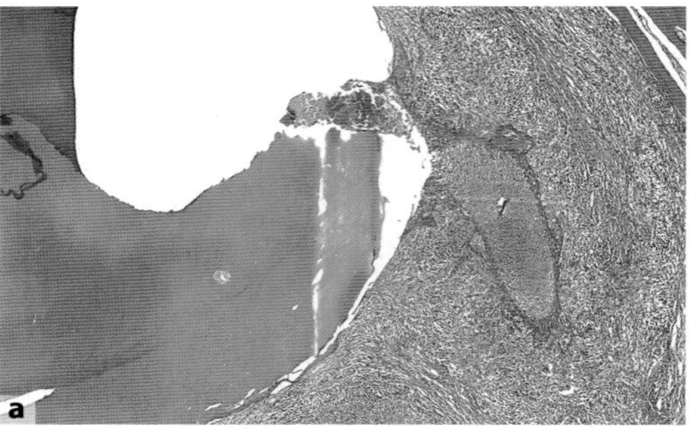

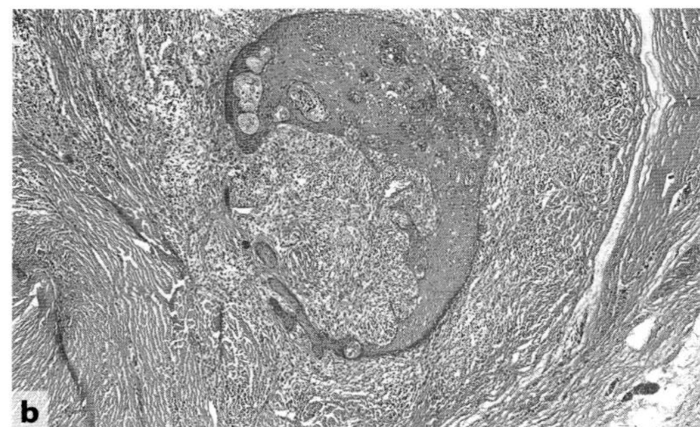

Fig. 9.3a,b Initial stage of radicular cyst. Epithelial proliferation in periapical abscess. **a** Overview with root surface at left side. **b** Higher magnification to show epithelial nest embedded in infiltrate of neutrophilic granulocytes

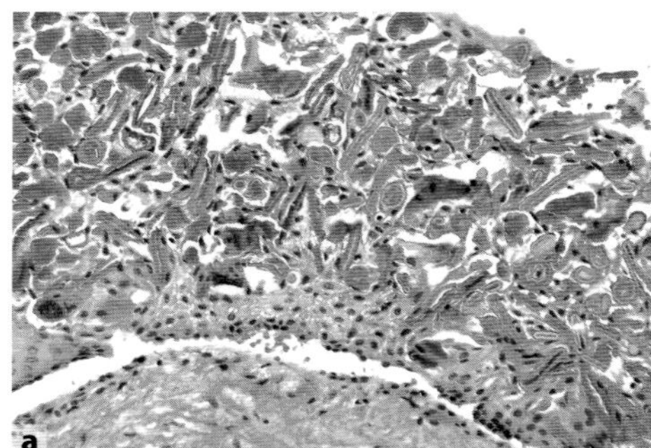

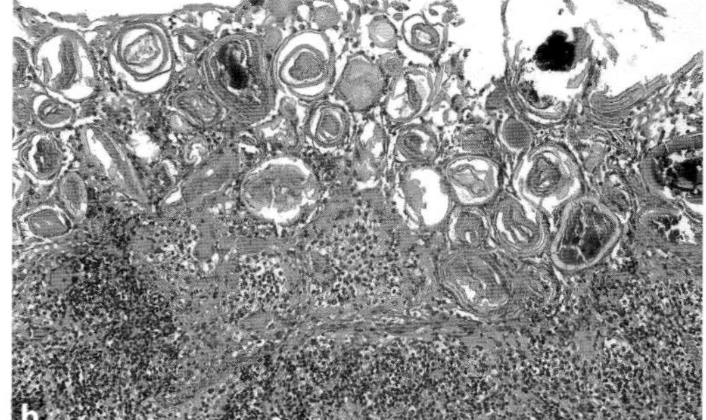

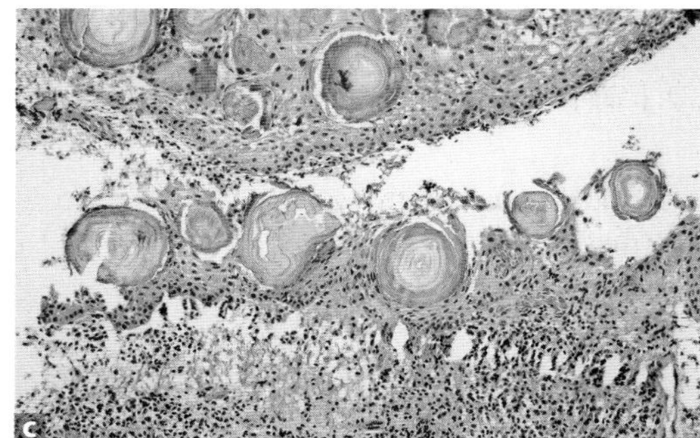

Fig. 9.4a–c Various appearances of Rushton bodies in epithelial lining of radicular cysts. **a** Rod-like, **b**, **c** More or less organised concentrically lamellated bodies

The specific nature of these so-called Rushton bodies is unclear [13]. Occasionally, the lining squamous cells are admixed with mucous cells or ciliated cells. Sometimes, the histologic pattern of the radicular cyst is complicated by extensive intramural proliferation of squamous epithelial nests of varying size, thus mimicking a squamous odontogenic tumour (Figs. 9.5a, b) [23] (see Sect. 10.1.4.).

The histologic appearance of the radicular cyst is rather unspecific. The same pattern may appear with other jaw cysts, especially the dentigerous cyst, in particular when the picture is dominated by inflammatory changes, thus obscuring the more specific features of the other cyst types. However, the clinical presentation, location at the root tip of a nonvital tooth, leaves little room for other diagnostic possibilities.

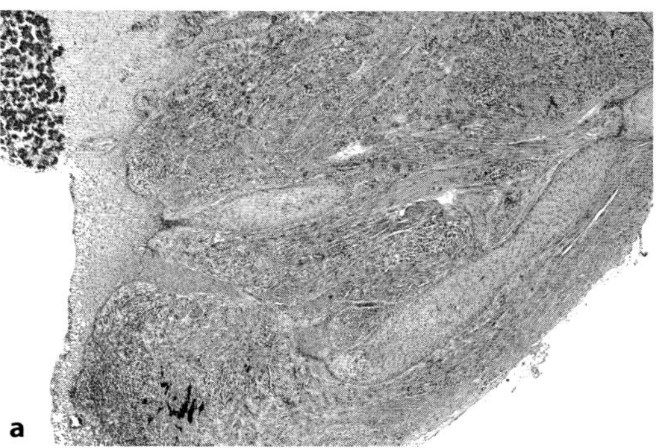

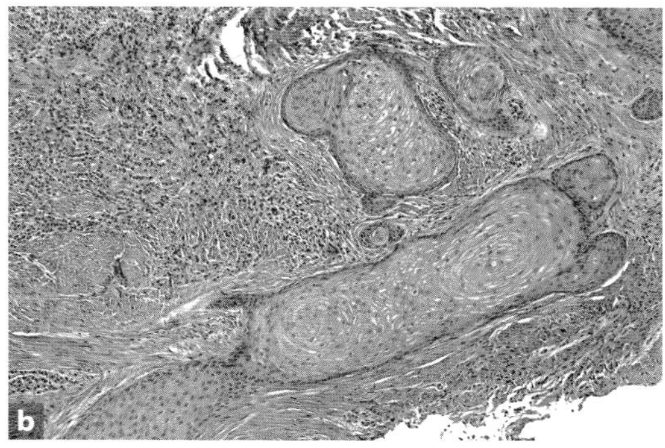

Fig. 9.5a,b Intramural epithelial proliferation in wall of radicular cyst. **a** Overview and **b** Detail. This may mimic squamous odontogenic tumour

When complicated by inflammation, radicular cysts may be characterised by pain and swelling. However, they may also be asymptomatic and only detected by radiographic examination of the dentition. In those cases, one sees a radiolucency at the root tip of a tooth. In case of additional lateral root foramina, the cyst may also lie in a lateral position. Tooth extraction or apical resection with curettage of the periapex usually is adequate treatment.

9.1.2 Residual Cyst

A residual cyst is nothing else than a radicular cyst that is retained in the jaws after removal of the associated tooth. Mostly, the inflammatory alterations and the ensuing epithelial proliferation are less prominent than in the radicular cyst. There are no other specific items different from the radicular cyst that would justify extensive separate discussion of this cyst type.

9.1.3 Paradental Cyst

Paradental cysts are located at the lateral side of the tooth at the border between enamel and root cementum (Fig. 9.6). They are secondary to an inflammatory process in the adjacent periodontal tissues that induces proliferation of neighbouring odontogenic epithelial rests, similar to the pathogenesis of the radicular cyst [10]. Histologically, they resemble the other inflammatory odontogenic cysts, the distinction being made by their specific clinical presentation and the vitality of the involved tooth. They are rare lesions, accounting for less than 3% in major series [18]. Treatment consists of excision with or without concomitant extraction of the involved tooth [4, 17].

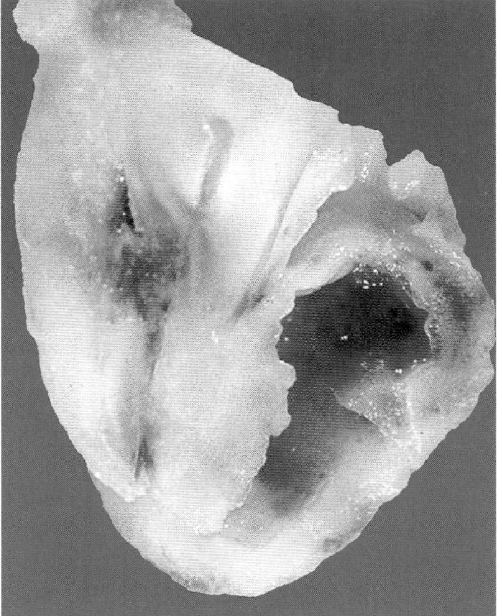

Fig. 9.6 Gross appearance of paradental cyst. Cystic cavity lying lateral to root surface

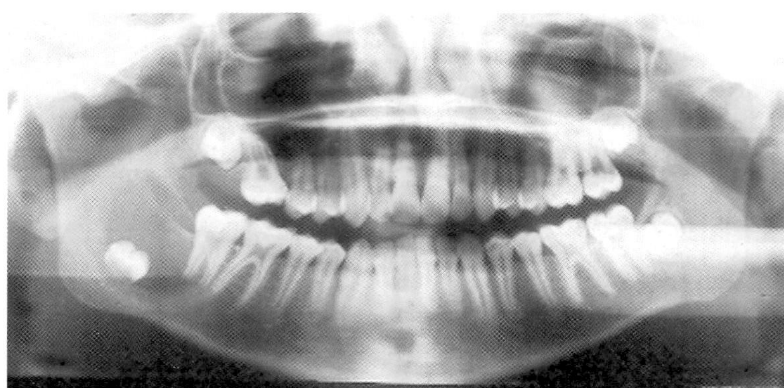

Fig. 9.7 Radiograph showing dentigerous cyst. In the right mandible, an impacted tooth can be seen to be surrounded by a unilocular radiolucency

9.2 Odontogenic Cysts—Developmental

9.2.1 Dentigerous Cyst

A dentigerous cyst (synonymous term follicular cyst) is a cyst that surrounds the crown of an unerupted tooth and is attached to the neck of this tooth (Fig. 9.7).

Dentigerous cysts are quite common. In larger series [18], they comprise almost 17% of all cases, only surpassed by radicular cysts. In most instances, they are associated with the maxillary canine or the mandibular third molar tooth.

Dentigerous cysts probably develop by accumulation of fluid between the reduced enamel epithelium and the crown surface or between the layers of the enamel epithelium itself [9]. Therefore, in contrast with the inflammatory cysts, no epithelial proliferation is needed to form this cyst.

When removed in toto, one sees a bag from which the root part of the involved tooth protrudes (Fig. 9.8). Opening of the bag discloses the crown of the tooth, the cyst bag forming a

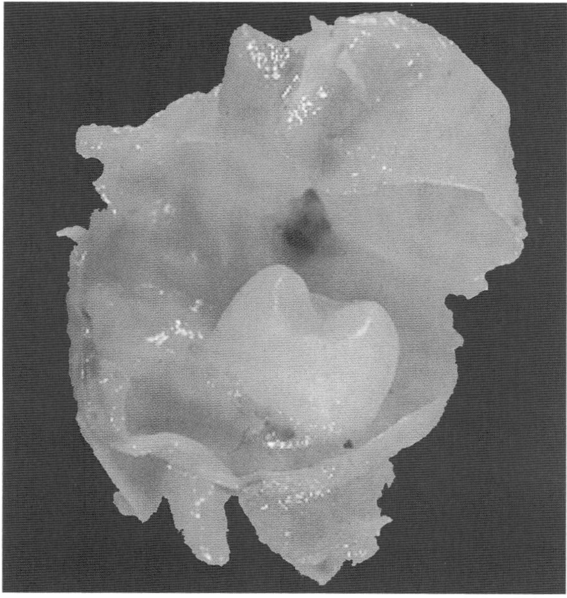

Fig. 9.8 Gross appearance of dentigerous cyst: tooth crown surrounded by thin-walled cyst that is attached to the neck of the involved tooth

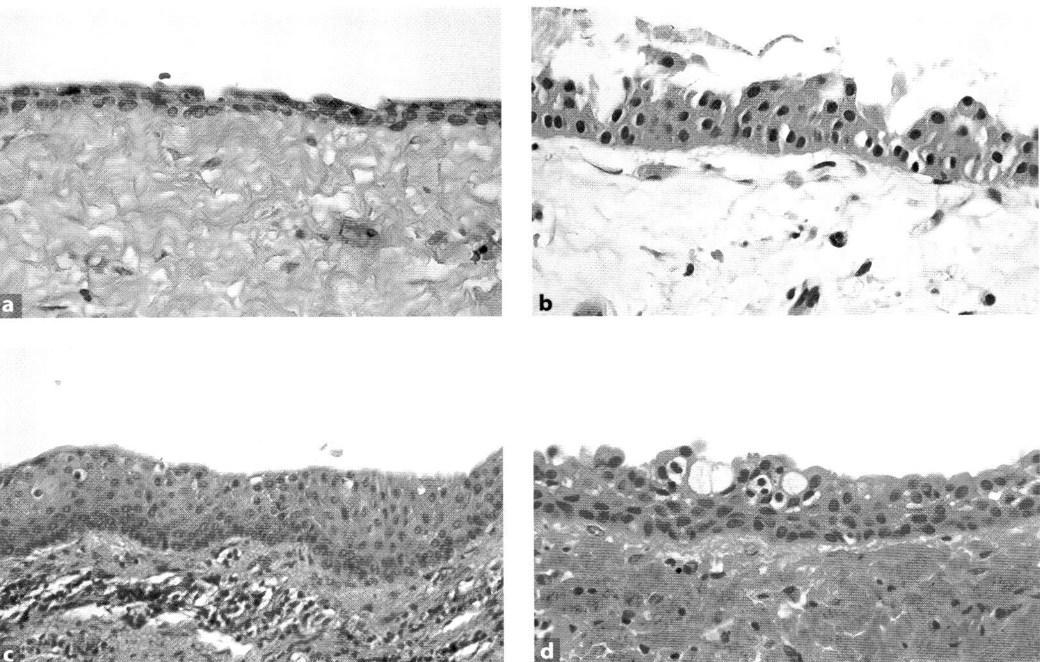

Fig. 9.9a–d Various appearances of epithelial lining in dentigerous cysts. **a** Most simple pattern consisting of two-layered cuboidal epithelium. **b** Cuboidal cells with interspersed columnar cells reminiscent of the columnar cells of the inner enamel epithelium. **c** Nonkeratinised squamous epithelium usually occurring if there is an inflammatory infiltrate in the underlying stroma. **d** Mucous cells lying between squamous cells

collar at the neck of the tooth. Usually, however, the tooth is separated from the soft tissue during the surgical removal and then no specific macroscopic features can be recognised.

Histologically, the cyst wall has a thin epithelial lining that may be only two to three cells thick and which resembles the reduced enamel epithelium (Fig. 9.9a). Sometimes, the original columnar shape of the cells of the inner enamel epithelium can still be recognised (Fig. 9.9b). In case of inflammation, the epithelium becomes thicker and will show features similar to the lining of a radicular cyst (Fig. 9.9c). Also, mucus-producing cells as well as ciliated cells may be observed (Fig. 9.9d). The connective tissue component of the cyst wall may be fibrous or fibromyxomatous. The cyst wall may also contain varying amounts of epithelial nests representing remnants of the dental lamina. If the relationship between involved tooth and cyst bag is uncompromised, the cyst wall can be seen to be attached to the tooth surface at the level of the cemento-enamel junction (Fig. 9.10).

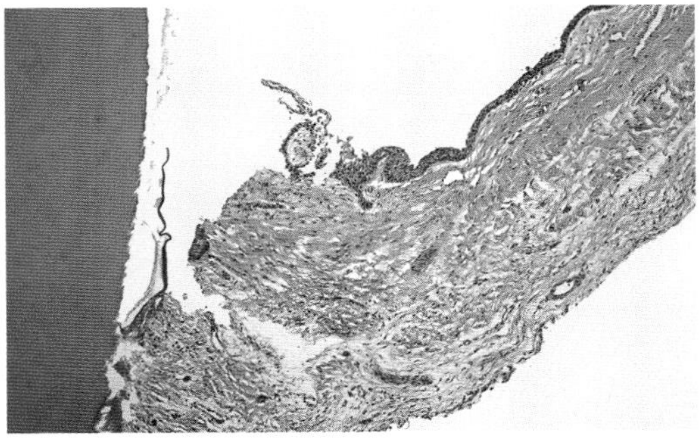

Fig. 9.10 Dentigerous cyst wall attached to the root surface at the level of the cemento-enamel junction (*left side*)

Radiologically, many jaw diseases associated with unerupted teeth may show an appearance similar the one shown by a dentigerous cyst. Histologic examination, however, will be decisive in ruling out these possibilities among which keratocystic odontogenic tumour and unicystic ameloblastoma (see Sects. 10.1.1, 10.1.5) are the most prevalent. Moreover, the radiologic picture of the dentigerous cyst may be mimicked by hyperplasia of the dental follicle, the connective tissue capsule that surrounds the unerupted tooth. This diagnostic dilemma can only be solved by surgery, in which case encountering either a cystic cavity or a soft tissue mass will reveal the real nature of the radiolucency surrounding the crown of the unerupted tooth [2].

Fibromyxomatous areas in the connective tissue wall of the dentigerous cyst may resemble odontogenic myxoma (see Sect. 10.2.1). Presence of odontogenic epithelial rests may lead to the erroneous diagnosis of one or another type of epithelial odontogenic tumour [8]. However, identification of the epithelial cyst lining will rule out these alternatives and lead to the appropriate diagnosis.

In case of excessive inflammatory changes, the histologic appearance of the dentigerous cyst is similar to the radicular cyst. Then only clinical information about the relationship between cyst and involved tooth and radiological appearance will enable the correct diagnosis: a radiolucent lesion surrounding the crown of an impacted tooth in case of a dentigerous cyst and a radiolucency at the root tip of an erupted nonvital tooth in case of a radicular cyst.

In most instances, dentigerous cysts will be a fortuitous finding on oral radiographs. Only when excessively large, may they cause swelling of the involved part of the jaw. In case of inflammation, pain and swelling will draw attention to the underlying cause. Removal of the cyst wall and the involved tooth will yield a permanent cure.

The *eruption cyst* is a specific type of dentigerous cyst located in the gingival soft tissues overlying the crown of an erupting tooth. Clinically, they appear as blue-stained blisters of the oral mucosa, the blood-stained cyst content being visible through the thin membrane separating cyst content from oral cavity (Fig. 9.11). Mostly, these cysts are short-lived, rupturing with progressive eruption of the associated tooth. Histologically, these cysts are lined by squamous epithelium that is thickened due to inflammatory changes in the underlying connective tissue and thus similar to the lining of a radicular cyst.

9.2.2 Lateral Periodontal Cyst

Lateral periodontal cysts occur at the lateral aspect or between the roots of vital teeth. They arise

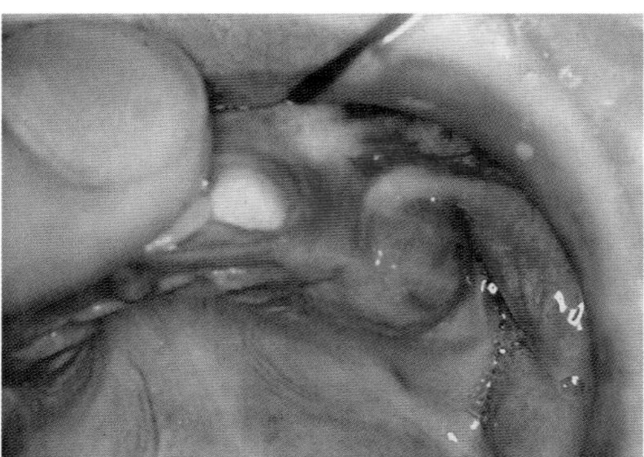

Fig. 9.11 Eruption cyst shimmering blue through its thin covering membrane

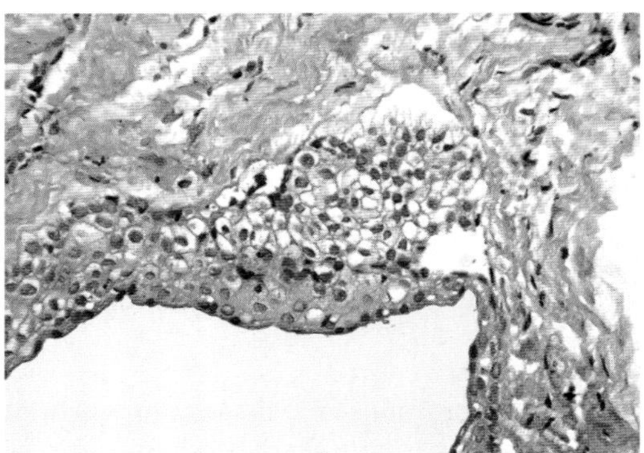

Fig. 9.12 Lateral periodontal cyst showing cuboidal epithelium thickening to form a plaque composed of clear cells

from odontogenic epithelial remnants: fragments of the dental lamina, reduced enamel epithelium, or rests of Malassez [21]. Inflammation does not play a role in their development.

The cyst is lined by a thin, nonkeratinising squamous or cuboidal epithelium with a thickness varying from one to five cell layers. Its most typical feature are focal, plaque-like thickenings that consist of clear cells that may contain glycogen (Fig. 9.12) [19]. The underlying connective tissue does not show prominent inflammatory changes.

The lateral periodontal cyst may be confused with other cysts that may lie lateral to the root of the tooth. The most important of them is a radicular cyst not occurring at the root tip but at the opening of an accessory canal. However, in case of lateral periodontal cysts, the involved tooth is vital and in case of radicular cysts by definition not. Moreover, acknowledging the specific histology of the lateral periodontal cyst will allow separation from the radicular cyst. The same histology serves to distinguish the lateral periodontal cyst from other cystic or solid lesions that may manifest themselves as paradental radiolucencies.

Lateral periodontal cysts do not cause any symptoms. They are fortuitous findings on radiographs where they present themselves as a well-demarcated radiolucency on the lateral surface of a tooth root. Simple enucleation is adequate treatment.

9.2.3 Botryoid Odontogenic Cyst

The botryoid odontogenic cyst represents a multilocular form of the lateral periodontal cyst with the same clinical and histologic appearance. Only a limited number of cases of this entity have been reported [7]. Treatment by curettage is the most appropriate treatment but recurrences may occur, sometimes after a long time interval [6].

9.2.4 Glandular Odontogenic Cyst

Glandular odontogenic cyst, also called sialo-odontogenic cyst, represents a cystic lesion that is characterised by an epithelial lining with cuboidal or columnar cells both at the surface and lining crypts or cyst-like spaces within the thickness of the epithelium [9, 16].

The lesion is very rare, accounting for only 0.04% in a large series of jaw cysts [3].

The lining epithelium partly consists of nonkeratinising squamous epithelium of varying thickness with focal thickenings similar to the plaques in the lateral periodontal cyst and the botryoid odontogenic cyst. This stratified epithelium may have a surface layer of eosinophilic cuboidal or columnar cells that can have cilia and sometimes form papillary projections.

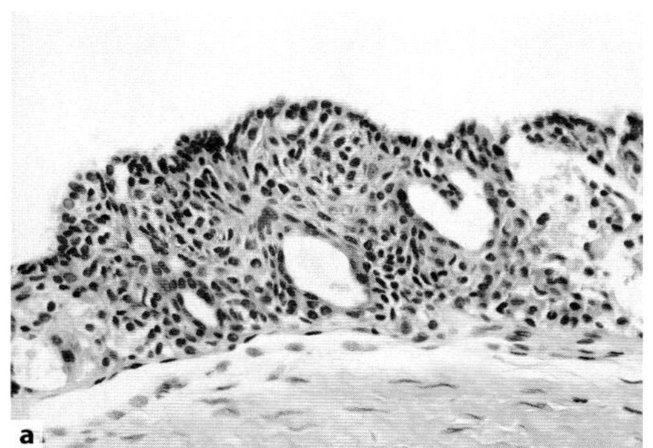

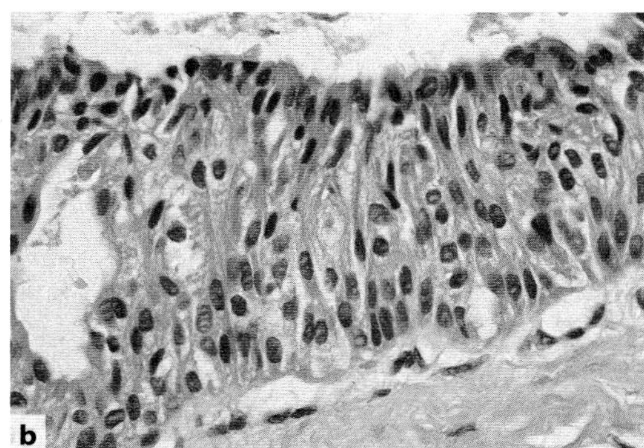

Fig. 9.13a,b Sialo-odontogenic cyst. **a** Overview showing epithelial lining containing ductal lumina. **b** Higher magnification to show some whorling of the epithelium and the low columnar nature of the most superficial epithelial layer

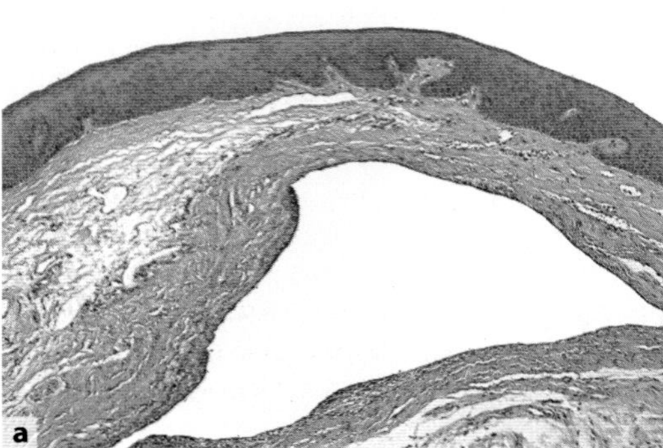

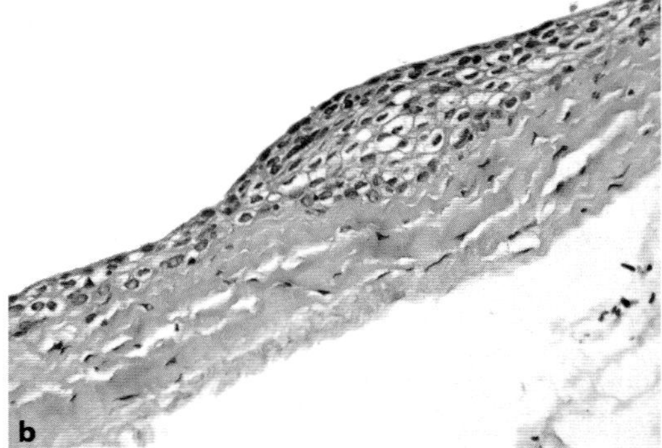

Fig. 9.14a,b Gingival cyst. **a** Low power view to show relationship between cyst lumen and overlying oral mucosal lining. **b** Cyst lining increasing in size and forming a plaque consisting of clear cells similar to those in the lateral periodontal cyst

Some of these superficial cells may assume an apocrine appearance with cytoplasmic fragments budding off into the cyst lumen. Also, mucus-producing cells may be present, either at the epithelial surface or as clusters within the epithelial lining. Focally, the epithelium shows areas of increased thickness in which glandular spaces form which may be lined by the various above mentioned cell types (Figs. 9.13a, b). Focally, the epithelial cells may be arranged into spherical structures with a whorled appearance.

Mucous cells and cuboidal cells with cilia may occur in many other jaw cysts, in particular in the dentigerous cyst. Therefore, in the absence of the other histologic features, their mere presence should not lead to the diagnosis of glandular odontogenic cyst.

Mucoepidermoid carcinoma is the major alternative that should be considered. The combination of nonkeratinising squamous epithelium and mucus-producing cells also characterises this salivary gland neoplasm that may occur intraosseously [11, 22]. However, epithelial plaques consisting of clear cells are not a feature of this latter lesion. When they are not found, it may be impossible to make the distinction.

The glandular odontogenic cyst most commonly affects the body of the mandible and the most prominent symptom is painless swelling. Treatment may be conservative but recurrence may occur [5].

9.2.5 Primordial Cyst

Primordial cysts are ill-defined lesions. Initially, the term was used for cystic lesions that were thought to arise through cystic degeneration of the very immature enamel organ, and thus replacing a tooth. Later, the term was also employed to define the lesion formerly called odontogenic keratocyst but currently known as keratocystic odontogenic tumour [15] (see Sect. 10.1.5).

9.2.6 Gingival Cyst

Gingival cysts are divided in those occurring in adults and in infants. Both, as the name already implies, are located in the gingival tissues. *Gingival cysts of adults* are rarely larger than 1 cm. They may be multiple. Possibly they arise from dental lamina rests. Histologically, they are lined by thin epithelium of one to three cell layers. This epithelium may also be thicker and exhibiting keratinisation. Plaques similar to those occurring in the lateral periodontal cyst may be seen (Figs. 9.14a, b) [14]. Possibly, both lesions are the same, only differing in location.

Gingival cysts of infants occur either as single or multiple cysts on the edentulous alveolar ridge of the newborn infant. When occurring at the midpalatal raphe, they are known as *palatal cysts of infants.* These tiny lesions, usually not larger than 3 mm, arise from dental lamina rests and disappear spontaneously within a short time. Histologically, they resemble epidermoid cysts [1, 12]. Historically, Epstein's pearls and Bohn's nodules are terms that have been used for these lesions.

References

1. Cataldo E, Berkman MD (1968) Cysts of the oral mucosa in newborns. Am J Dis Child 16:44–48
2. Daley TD, Wysocki GP (1995) The small dentigerous cyst. Oral Surg Oral Med Oral Pathol Oral Radiol Endod 79:77–81
3. Daley TD, Wysocki GP, Pringle GA (1994) Relative incidence of odontogenic tumors and oral and jaw cysts in a Canadian population. Oral Surg Oral Med Oral Pathol 77:276–280
4. Fowler CB, Brannon RB (1989) The paradental cyst: a clinicopathologic study of six new cases and review of the literature. J Oral Maxillofac Surg 47:243–248
5. Gardner DG, Morency R (1993) The glandular odontogenic cyst; a rare lesion that tends to recur. J Can Dent Assoc 59:929–930
6. Greer RO, Johnson M (1988) Botryoid odontogenic cyst: clinicopathologic analysis of ten cases with three recurrences. J Oral Maxillofac Surg 46:574–579
7. Gurol M, Burkes EJ, Jacoway J (1995) Botryoid odontogenic cyst: analysis of 33 cases. J Periodontol 66:1069–1073
8. Kim J, Ellis GL (1993) Dental follicular tissue: misinterpretation as odontogenic tumors. J Oral Maxillofac Surg 51:762–767
9. Kramer IRH, Pindborg JJ, Shear M (1992) Histological typing of odontogenic tumours. 2nd edn. Springer, Berlin. pp 10–42
10. Magnusson B, Borrman H (1995) The paradental cyst: a clinicopathologic study of 26 cases. Swed Dent J 19:1–7
11. Manojlovic S, Grguveric J, Knezevic G, Kruslin B (1997) Glandular odontogenic cyst: a case report and clinicopathologic analysis of the relationship to central mucoepidermoid carcinoma. Head Neck 19:227–231
12. Monteleone L, McLellan MS (1964) Epstein's pearls (Bohn's nodules) of the palate. J Oral Surg 22: 301–304
13. Morgan PR, Johnson NW (1974) Histological, histochemical and ultrastructural studies on the nature of hyaline bodies in odontogenic cysts. J Oral Pathol 3:127–147
14. Nxumalo TN, Shear M (1992) Gingival cysts in adults. J Oral Pathol Med 21:309–313
15. Philipsen HP (2005) Keratocystic odontogenic tumour. In: Barnes L, Eveson JW, Reichart PA, et al. (eds) World Health Organization Classification of Tumours. Pathology and genetics of tumours of the head and neck. IARC, Lyon. pp 306–307
16. Ramer M, Montazem A, Lane SL, Lumerman H (1997) Glandular odontogenic cyst. Report of a case and review of the literature. Oral Surg Oral Med Oral Pathol Oral Radiol Endod 84:54–57
17. Reichart PA, Philipsen HP (2003) Entzündliche paradentale Zyste. Bericht von 6 Fällen. Mund Kiefer Gesichtschir 7:171–174
18. Shear M (1992) Cysts of the oral regions. 3rd edn. Wright, Oxford. p 6
19. Shear M, Pindborg JJ (1975) Microscopic features of the lateral periodontal cyst. Scand J Dent Res 83:103–110
20. Slootweg PJ (2006) Chapter 4. Maxillofacial skeleton and teeth. In: Cardesa A, Slootweg PJ (eds.) Pathology of the head and neck. Springer, Heidelberg. pp 104–130
21. Suljak JP, Bohay RN, Wysocki GP (1998) Lateral periodontal cyst: a case report and review of the literature. J Can Dent Assoc 64:48–51
22. Waldron CA, Koh ML (1990) Central mucoepidermoid carcinoma of the jaws: report of four cases with analysis of the literature and discussion of the relationship to mucoepidermoid, sialodontogenic and glandular odontogenic cysts. J Oral Maxillofac Surg 48:871–877
23. Wright JM (1979) Squamous odontogenic tumorlike proliferations in odontogenic cysts. Oral Surg Oral Med Oral Pathol 47:354–358

Chapter 10

Odontogenic Tumours

10

Odontogenic tumours are comprised of a group of lesions which have in common the fact that they arise from the odontogenic tissue. They develop from the epithelial part of the tooth germ, the ectomesenchymal part, or from both. Their behaviour varies from frankly neoplastic, including metastatic potential, to nonneoplastic hamartomatous. Some of them may recapitulate normal tooth development, including the formation of dental hard tissues such as enamel, dentin, and cementum [9, 10, 15].

10.1 Epithelial

Epithelial odontogenic tumours are supposed to be derived from odontogenic epithelium: dental lamina, enamel organ, and Hertwig's root sheath. As there is no contribution, either proliferative or inductive, from the odontogenic mesenchyme, these lesions do not contain dental hard tissues or myxoid tissue resembling the dental papilla.

10.1.1 Ameloblastoma

Ameloblastomas closely resemble the epithelial part of the tooth germ. They behave aggressively locally, but do not metastasise. It is the most common odontogenic tumour (Fig. 10.1a) [2, 12].

Ameloblastomas consist of either anastomosing epithelial strands and fields or discrete epithelial islands. The former pattern is called the *plexiform* type, the other the *follicular* (Figs. 10.1b, c). Both may occur within one and the same lesion. The peripheral cells at the border with the adjacent fibrous stroma are columnar, with nuclei usually in the apical half of the cell body away from the basement membrane. The cells lying

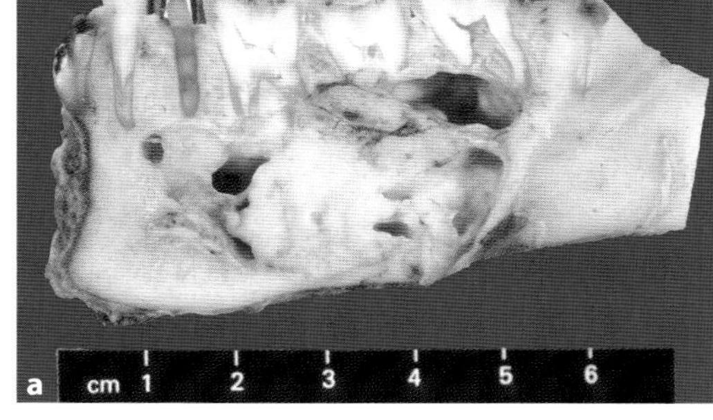

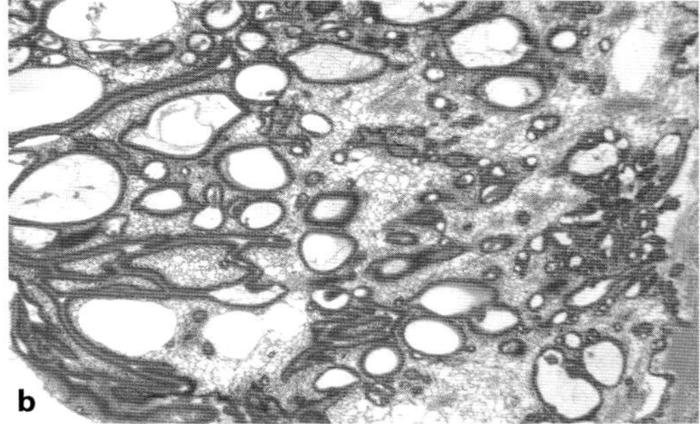

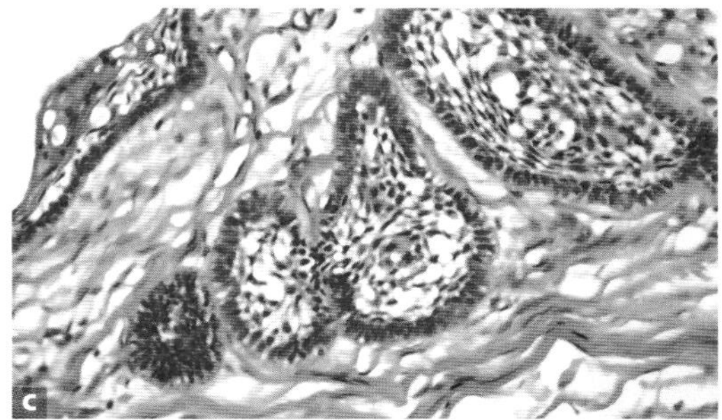

Fig. 10.1 **a** Cut surface showing gross appearance of ameloblastoma. Note destruction of jaw bone and external resorption of the involved tooth roots. Photomicrograph showing plexiform (**b**) and follicular (**c**) type ameloblastoma. Especially the epithelial nests in the follicular type show close similarity to the enamel organ of the tooth germ in the cap and bell stage. Compare with Fig. 1.3

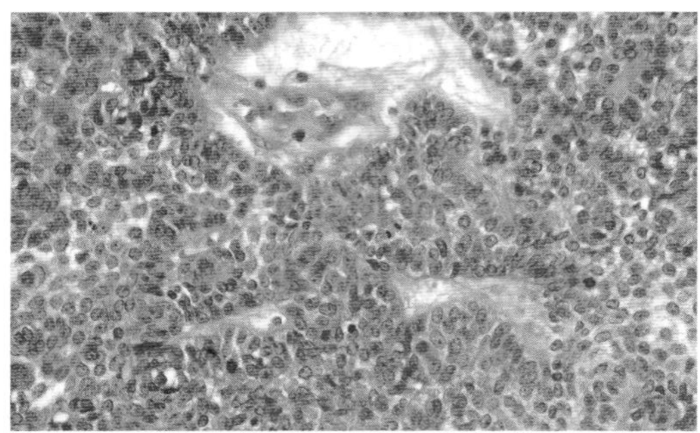

Fig. 10.2 Mitotic activity in an ameloblastoma without cytonuclear atypia. This feature should not be interpreted to indicate malignancy

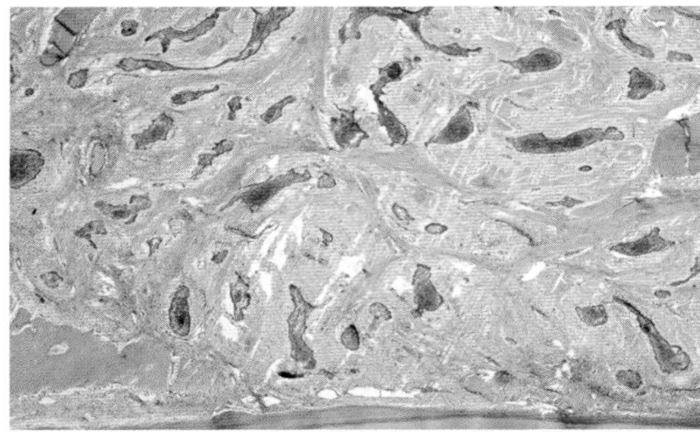

Fig. 10.3 In desmoplastic ameloblastoma, the resemblance to the enamel organ is less obvious

more centrally are fusiform to polyhedral and loosely connected to each other through cytoplasmic extensions. At the periphery of the lesion, the tumour infiltrates into the adjacent cancellous bone. The lower cortical border of the mandible and the periosteal layer usually expand, but will not be perforated, the periosteum in particular forming a barrier [11]. Spread into soft tissues is highly unusual; a tumour combining this feature with an ameloblastic appearance probably is an ameloblastic carcinoma (see Sect. 10.4.2). Mitotic figures may occur within the peripheral columnar as well as in the stellate reticulum-like cells (Fig. 10.2). In the absence of cytonuclear atypia and with a normal configuration, they are without prognostic significance.

Acanthomatous and *granular cell* type ameloblastoma are variants of follicular ameloblastoma with squamous metaplasia and granular cells, respectively. If keratinisation is abundant, leading to large cavities filled with keratin, lesions are called *keratoameloblastoma.* In these tumours, acantholysis may lead to a pseudopapillary lining that characterises the variant called *papilliferous keratoameloblastoma.* The *basal cell (basaloid) ameloblastoma* is composed of nests of basaloid cells with a peripheral rim of cuboidal cells and does not display a well-developed, loose oedematous centre. *Desmoplastic ameloblastoma* shows a dense collagenous stroma, the epithelial component being reduced to narrow, compressed strands of epithelium. When these strands broaden to form larger islands, a peripheral rim of dark staining cuboidal cells and a compact centre in which spindle-shaped epithelial cells assume a whorling pattern may be discerned (Fig. 10.3). Within the stromal component, active bone formation can be observed. *Unicystic ameloblastoma* represents a cyst that is lined by ameloblastomatous epithelium [12]. This epithelium may proliferate to form intraluminal nodules with the architecture of plexiform ameloblastoma. Downward proliferation of this epithelium may lead to infiltration of the fibrous cyst wall by ameloblastoma nests. Sometimes, the cyst lining itself lacks any features indicative of ameloblastoma, these being confined to intramural epithelial nests [12]. Inflammatory alterations may obscure the specific histologic details to such an extent that none are left. Unicystic ameloblastomas in which the ameloblastomatous epithelium only lines the cystic surface can be treated in a more limited way than those in which there is also epithelial downgrowth into the fibrous cyst wall. The latter have to be treated in the same way as the conventional solid and multicystic ameloblastomas and require removal including a rim of surrounding tissues.

Epithelial nests resembling ameloblastoma may be found in ameloblastic fibromas and calcifying odontogenic cysts, lesions to be discussed under the appropriate headings (see Sects. 10.3.1, 10.3.6). Also, epithelial nests in the dental follicle that surrounds an impacted tooth and in the wall of odontogenic cysts may mimic ameloblastoma [5, 14].

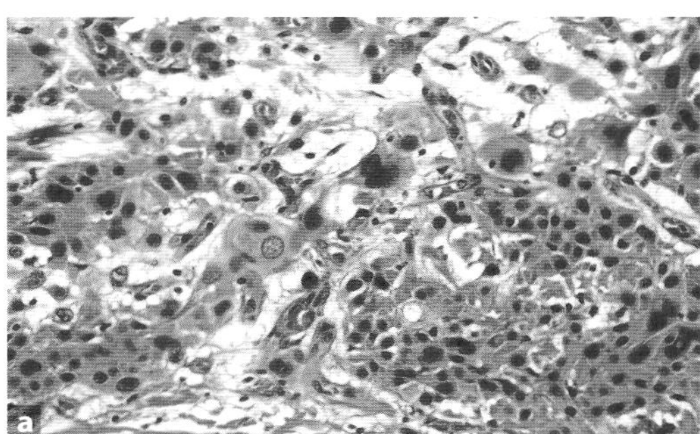

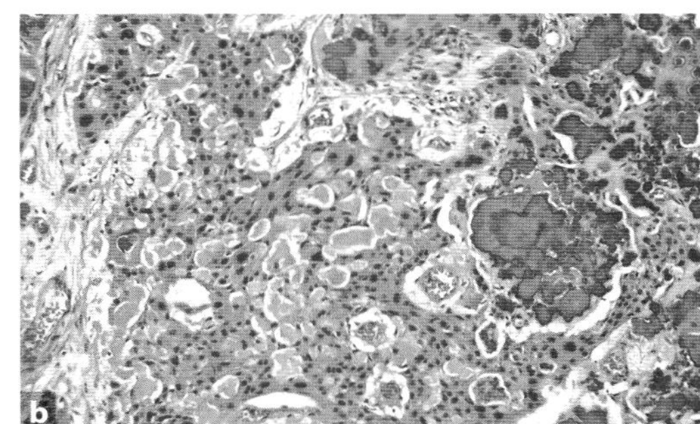

Fig. 10.4a,b Calcifiying epithelial odontogenic tumour. Nuclear pleomorphism is clearly displayed (**a**). Note also the concentrically lamellated calcified particles (**b**)

Sometimes, ameloblastomas present themselves as soft tissue swellings occurring in the tooth-bearing areas of the maxilla or mandible without involvement of the underlying bone. This *peripheral ameloblastoma* should not be confused with intraosseous ameloblastomas that spread from within the jaw into the overlying gingiva.

10.1.2 Calcifying Epithelial Odontogenic Tumour

The calcifying epithelial odontogenic tumour consists of sheets of polygonal cells with ample eosinophilic cytoplasm, distinct cell borders, and very conspicuous intercellular bridges. Nuclei are pleomorphic with prominent nucleoli; cells with giant nuclei and multiple nuclei are also present. Mitotic figures, however, are absent. Clear cell differentiation may occur. The epithelial tumour islands as well as the surrounding stroma frequently contain concentrically lamellated calcifications. The stroma contains eosinophilic material that stains like amyloid (Figs. 10.4a, b). Also stromal deposits of bone and cementum may occur. There is no encapsulation. The tumour grows into the cancellous spaces of the adjacent jaw bone while causing expansion and thinning of the cortical bone. Sometimes an impacted tooth may be present centrally within the tumour mass (Fig. 10.5)

10.1.3 Adenomatoid Odontogenic Tumour

Grossly, the adenomatoid odontogenic tumour is a cyst that embraces the crown of the involved tooth (Fig. 10.6). The lesion consists of two different cell populations: spindle-shaped and columnar. The spindle-shaped cells form whorled nodules that may contain droplets of eosinophilic material. A lattice of thin epithelial strands usually connects these nodules to each other. The columnar cells line duct-like spaces with a lumen either empty or containing eosinophilic material, and may form curvilinear opposing rows with interposed eosinophilic material (Figs. 10.7a, b). In the stroma, there are large aggregates of eo-

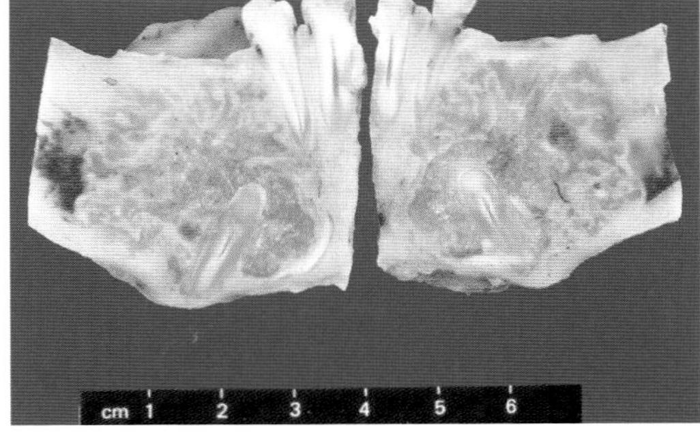

Fig. 10.5 Cut surface of jaw specimen with calcifying epithelial odontogenic tumour. The tumour surrounds an impacted tooth and is not encapsulated

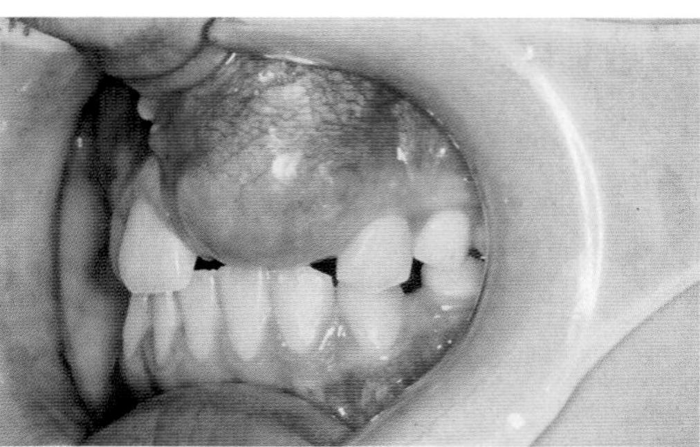

Fig. 10.6 Clinical appearance of adenomatoid odontogenic tumour. Cystic swelling occupies the jaw area where an incisor tooth should be present

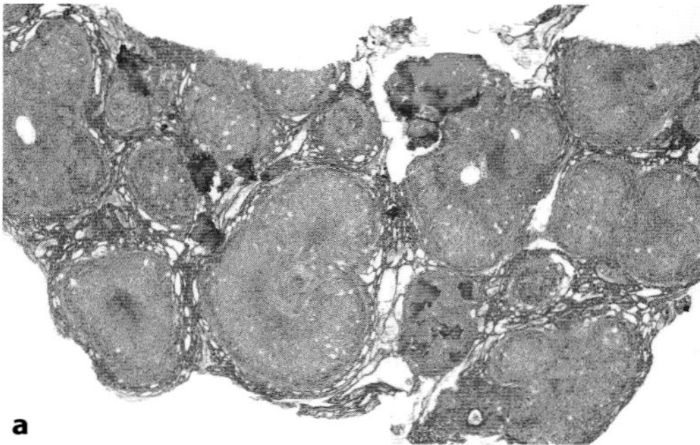

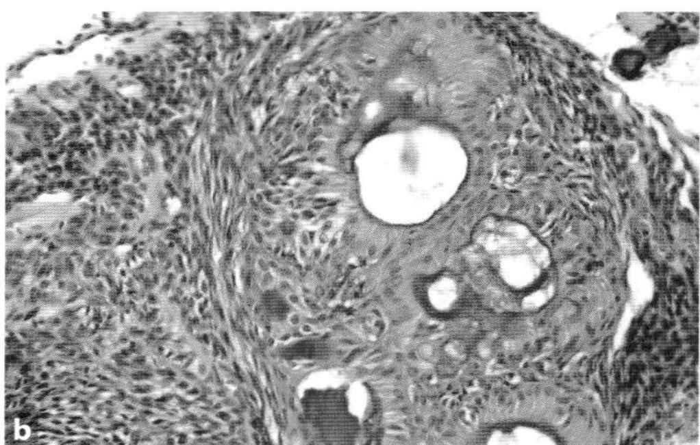

Fig. 10.7 Photomicrograph showing epithelial nests connected by epithelial strands as is typical for adenomatoid odontogenic tumour (**a**). At higher magnification, the alternation of spindle-cells and lumen-lining columnar cells can be observed (**b**)

sinophilic hyaline material, which is judged to be either a dysplastic form of dentin, cementum, or a metaplastic reaction of the stromal tissue. Also, concentrically laminated calcified bodies similar to those seen in calcifying epithelial odontogenic tumours may occur. In some adenomatoid odontogenic tumours, areas of eosinophilic cells with well-defined cell boundaries and prominent intercellular bridges similar to those observed in the calcifying epithelial odontogenic tumour are seen. They do not influence the biologic behaviour of this tumour and are considered to be part of its histologic spectrum.

10.1.4 Squamous Odontogenic Tumour

Squamous odontogenic tumour is composed of islands of well-differentiated squamous epithelium surrounded by mature fibrous connective tissue. There is no cellular atypia. There is spinous differentiation with well-defined intercellular bridges, but keratinisation is unusual. In the epithelial islands, cystic degeneration and calcification may

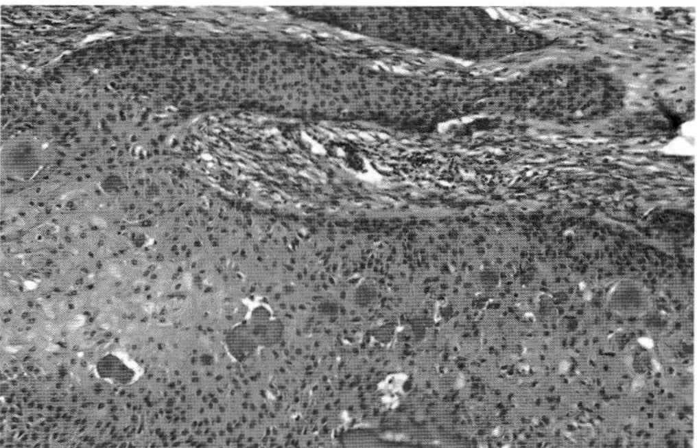

Fig. 10.8 Squamous odontogenic tumour consists of well-differentiated epithelial nests exhibiting squamous differentiation and calcification. Peripheral palissading indicative of ameloblastoma is lacking as is cytonuclear atypia seen in squamous cell carcinoma

occur (Fig. 10.8). Invasion into cancellous bone may be present. The absence of cytonuclear atypia rules out well-differentiated squamous cell carcinoma and the absence of peripheral palisading of columnar cells excludes ameloblastoma as alternative diagnosis. Sometimes, intramural epithelial proliferation in jaw cysts may simulate squamous odontogenic tumour (see Sect. 9.1.1). The lesion may cause loosening of the teeth involved.

10.1.5 Keratocystic Odontogenic Tumour

Keratocystic odontogenic tumour is more universally known as odontogenic keratocyst, but has been renamed as there is sufficient evidence that this lesion actually represents a cystic neoplasm [2, 12]. This lesion shows a thin connective tissue wall lined by stratified squamous epithelium with a well-defined basal layer of palisading columnar or cuboidal cells and with a superficial corrugated layer of parakeratin. Mitotic figures can be identified in parabasilar and midspinous areas. The underlying cyst wall may contain tiny daughter cysts and solid epithelial nests. Also, epithelial proliferations similar to ameloblastoma have been reported. When extensively inflamed, this lesion loses its typical histologic features, then only showing a nonkeratinising stratified epithelium exhibiting spongiosis and elongated rete pegs supported by a connective tissue containing a mixed inflammatory infiltrate (Figs. 10.9a–c). Multiple keratocystic odontogenic tumours occur within the context of the nevoid basal cell carcinoma syndrome [4].

10.2 Mesenchymal

Mesenchymal odontogenic tumours are derived from the ectomesenchymal part of the tissues

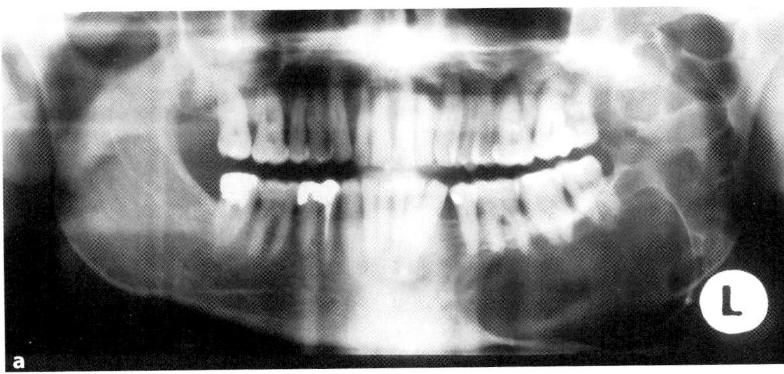

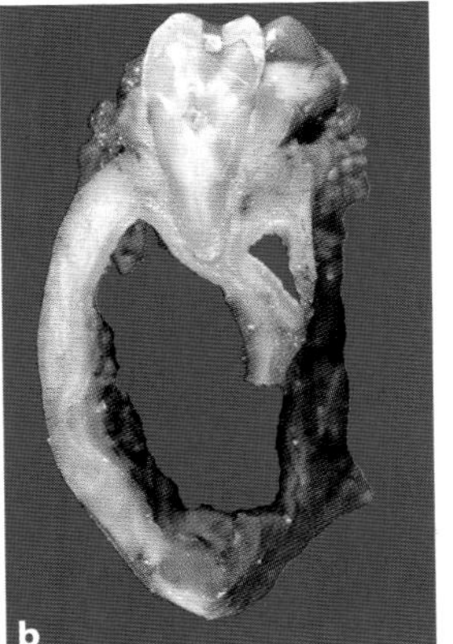

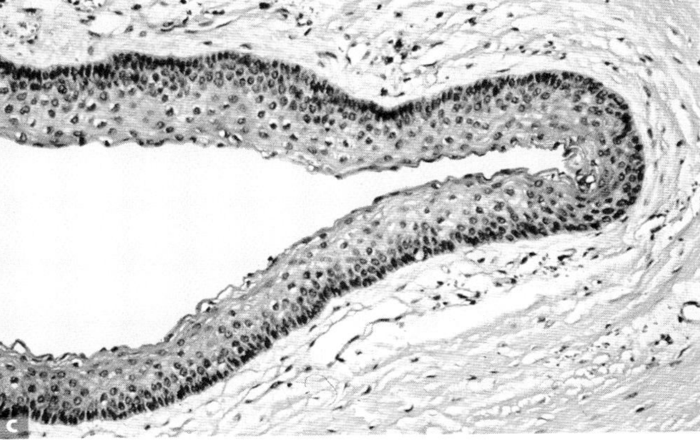

Fig. 10.9a–c Keratocystic odontogenic tumour. **a** Radiograph showing extensive bone loss in left mandible. **b** Slice from same mandible as shown in **a** to illustrate the way the lesion has hollowed out the mandible. **c** Photomicrograph showing cyst lining typically composed of columnar basal cells and a corrugated parakeratinising surface

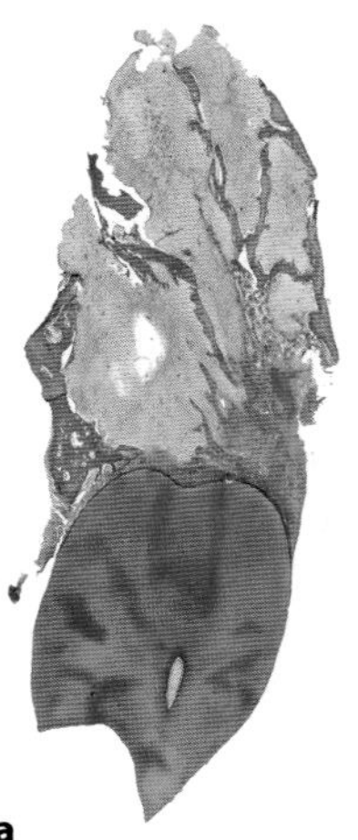

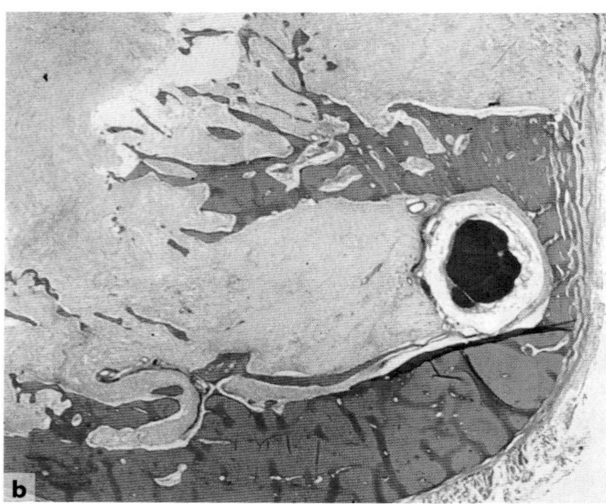

Fig. 10.10 Low (**a**) and intermediate (**b**) power view of myxoma. The lesion is composed of myxoid material engulfing cancellous jaw bone

that participate in the development of teeth and periodontal tissues. Odontogenic epithelial rests may be part of the histologic picture they show, but represent only structures fortuitously engulfed by tumour tissue. They have no neoplastic or inductive potential.

10.2.1 Odontogenic Myxoma

Odontogenic myxomas consist of rather monotonous cells with multipolar or bipolar slender cytoplasmic extensions that lie in a myxoid stroma. Nuclei vary from round to fusiform in appearance. Binucleated cells and mitotic figures are present, but scarce (Figs. 10.10a, b). Occasionally, the lesion contains odontogenic epithelial rests. They are a fortuitous finding without any diagnostic or prognostic significance. The lesion spreads into the jaw bone without any encapsulation, thereby engulfing neighbouring cancellous bone (Fig. 10.11).

Myxoma may be mimicked by dental follicle and dental papilla. Both contain myxoid areas [5, 8, 14]. Dental papilla tissue can be distinguished from myxoma by the presence of a peripheral layer of columnar odontoblasts. For both dental papilla and dental follicle, clinical and radiographic data are decisive in avoiding misinterpretation of myxomatous tissue in jaw specimens: in the first case, a tooth germ lies in the jaw area from which

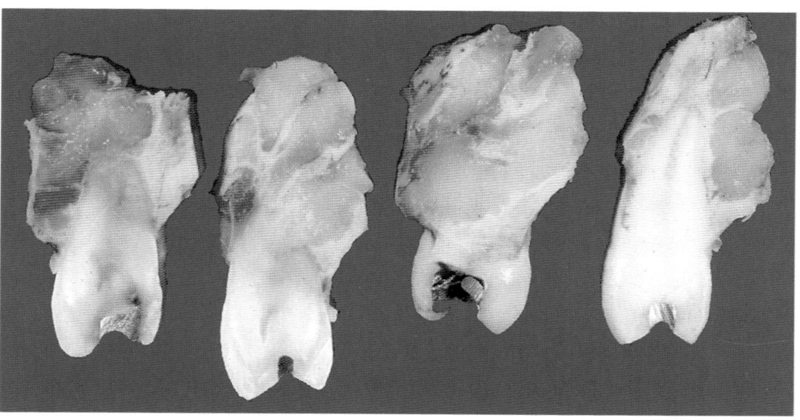

Fig. 10.11 The diffuse spread of the myxoma in the jaw bone is clearly displayed in the cut surface of this gross specimen of a maxillary myxoma

the submitted tissue has been taken, whereas in the second case, the tissue sample covered the crown area of an impacted tooth. This item will be discussed more extensively in Chap. 11.

10.2.2 Odontogenic Fibroma

Odontogenic fibroma is a controversial entity. Uncertainty exists about the broadness of the histologic spectrum that these lesions may show, and about its distinction from other fibrous jaw lesions [2, 12]. The lesion is seen within the jaw as well as in the gingiva (Fig. 10.12a). Odontogenic fibroma consists of fibroblasts lying in a background of myxoid material intermingled with collagen fibres that may vary from delicate to coarse (Fig. 10.12b). Odontogenic epithelium, either scarce or abundant, may occur. Only rarely is the epithelial component so conspicuous that differentiation between odontogenic fibroma and ameloblastoma may be difficult.

This histologic spectrum may expand to include cell-rich myxoid areas, a greater epithelial component, and varying amounts of amorphous calcified globules or mineralised collagenous matrix. Tumours with this more variegated histology have been referred to as *complex odontogenic fibroma* or *WHO-type odontogenic fibroma* [2]. Odontogenic fibroma may also contain granular cells. These lesions have been called granular cell odontogenic fibromas or, alternatively, granular cell ameloblastic fibromas. This tumour, however, could also represent a unique entity: *central odontogenic granular cell tumour* [3].

All histologic features shown by odontogenic fibroma may also be displayed by the dental follicle [5, 7]. In these cases, the radiographic appearance of the lesion, a small radiolucent rim surrounding the crown of a tooth buried within the jaw, will make the distinction (see also Chap. 11).

10.2.3 Cementoblastoma

Cementoblastomas are heavily mineralised cementum masses connected to the apical root part of a tooth (Fig. 10.13). They are composed of a vascular, loose-textured fibrous tissue that surrounds coarse trabeculae of basophilic mineralised material bordered by plump cells with ample cytoplasm and large but not atypical nuclei. Mitotic figures are rare. At the periphery, the mineralised material may form radiating spikes. Also, osteoclastic giant cells form part of the histologic spectrum. The hard tissue component is

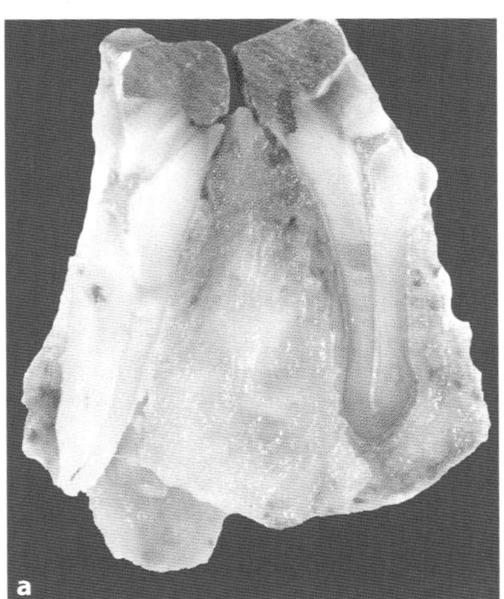

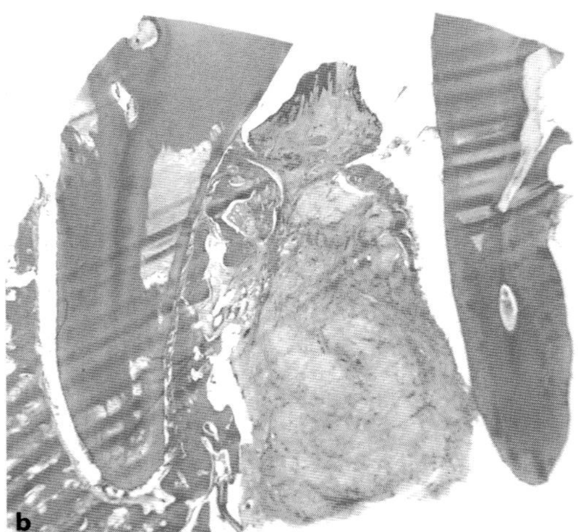

Fig. 10.12 a Cut surface of odontogenic fibroma situated between the roots of two adjacent teeth. It is this location that identifies the lesion as an odontogenic fibroma and not the histology that consists of fibrous tissue without any noteworthing features as shown in **b**

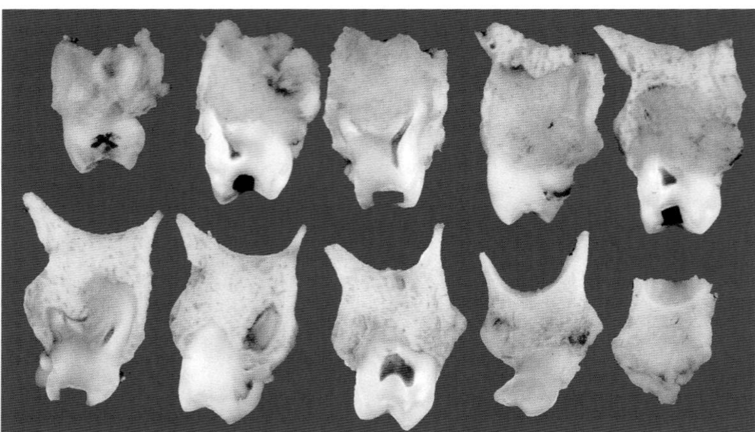

Fig. 10.13 Slices from a maxillary cementoblastoma. The hard tissue mass is connected to the roots of several maxillary teeth that show external resorption

connected with the root of the involved tooth, which usually shows signs of external resorption. The sharp border between the tubular dentin of the root and the hard tissue component forms the hallmark of cementoblastomas (Fig. 10.14).

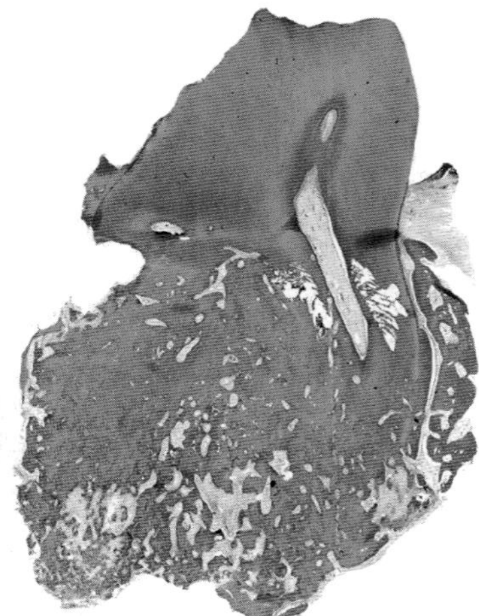

Fig. 10.14 Low power view of a cementoblastoma. The cementum-like material is continuous with the tooth roots that are partly resorbed. (From [13], with permission)

10.3 Odontogenic Tumours—Mixed Epithelial and Mesenchymal

Mixed odontogenic tumours are composed of both epithelial-derived and mesenchymal-derived tissues. These tumours recapitulate tissue proliferation and differentiation as seen in the developing teeth. Deposition of the dental hard tissues—enamel and dentin—may also occur. Lesions with an identical histology can show neoplastic as well as hamartomatous behaviour [2, 9, 12].

10.3.1 Ameloblastic Fibroma

Ameloblastic fibroma lacks a hard tissue component, only displaying soft tissues similar to those found in the immature tooth germ. The epithelial part of ameloblastic fibroma consists of branching and anastomosing epithelial strands that form knots of varying size. These knots have a peripheral rim of columnar cells that embraces a loosely arranged spindle-shaped epithelium. These epithelial strands lie in a myxoid cell-rich mesenchyme. The amount of epithelium may vary among cases and regionally within an individual case. There is no formation of dental hard tissues (Fig. 10.15). Mitotic figures, either in epithelium or mesenchyme, are extremely rare; when easily found, they should raise concern about the benign nature of the case. Ameloblastic fibroma may contain granular cells. Whether these le-

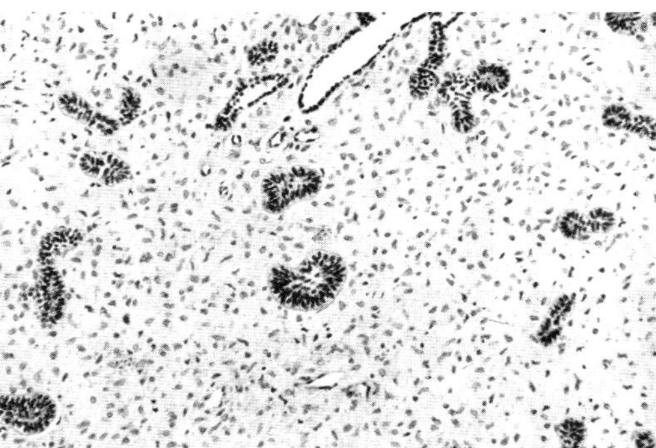

Fig. 10.15 Ameloblastic fibroma recapitulates the bud stage of the tooth germ. Epithelial strands forming buds containing palissading cylindrical cells at their periphery lie in a myxoid connective tissue similar to the mesenchymal cell condensation forming the presumptive dental papilla

sions should be called *granular cell ameloblastic fibroma* or *granular cell odontogenic fibroma* is controversial [3].

The epithelial component of ameloblastic fibroma closely resembles that of ameloblastoma. The stromal component, however, is entirely different: in ameloblastoma it is mature fibrous connective tissue whereas in the ameloblastic fibroma it is immature, embryonic, cell-rich myxoid tissue. Areas similar to ameloblastic fibroma may also be observed in the hyperplastic dental follicle [5, 14]. The radiographic appearance makes the distinction; a radiolucent rim surrounding an unerupted tooth in the case of a dental follicle and an expansive radiolucent jaw lesion in the case of an ameloblastic fibroma.

10.3.2 Ameloblastic Fibro-Odontoma

Ameloblastic fibro-odontomas are lesions that combine a soft tissue component, similar to ameloblastic fibroma, with the presence of dentin and enamel. In rare cases, only dentin is formed; those tumours are called *ameloblastic fibro-dentinoma* [9].

The soft tissue component is identical to that of ameloblastic fibroma. Dentin may be formed either as eosinophilic mineralised material containing tubuli, just as in normal teeth, but it may also form as an homogeneous eosinophilic mass with sparse cells included. It always lies in close association with adjacent epithelium and forms the scaffold for the deposition of enamel matrix that is laid down at the border between epithelium and dentin by columnar epithelial cells that have reached their terminal differentiation as ameloblasts. The dental hard tissues are arranged haphazardly without any reminiscence of the orderly structure characterising normal teeth (Fig. 10.16).

Hyperplastic dental follicles may also show focal areas with the appearance of ameloblastic fibro-odontoma. Differential diagnostic considerations are the same as those as already mentioned. Ameloblastic fibro-odontomas can be distinguished from ameloblastomas by the presence of cellular myxoid tissue and of dentin and enamel.

10.3.3 Odontoma—Complex Type

Complex odontomas consist of a usually well-delineated mass of dental hard tissues in a haphazard arrangement. The bulk of the lesion consists of dentin recognisable by the presence of tubuli. Enamel plays a minor role, usually confined to small rims in cavities in the dentin mass (Figs. 10.17a–e). The stroma consists of mature fibrous connective tissue. Sometimes, odontomas may contain areas identical to the calcifying odontogenic cyst, including ghost cells [16].

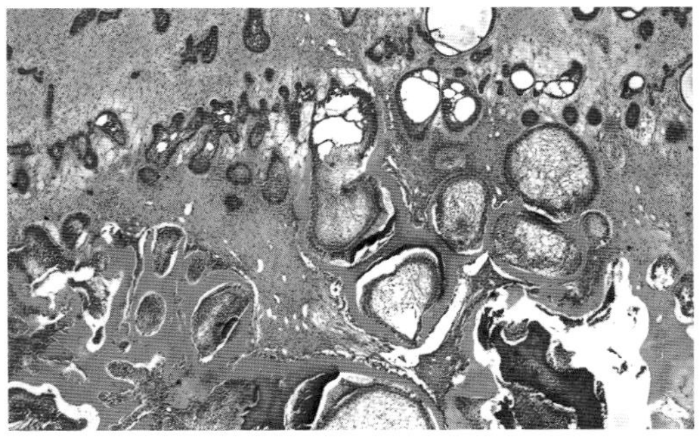

Fig. 10.16 Ameloblastic fibro-odontoma combines soft tissue component of ameloblastic fibroma with cell differentiation recapitulating the bell stage of the tooth germ with formation of dentin and enamel

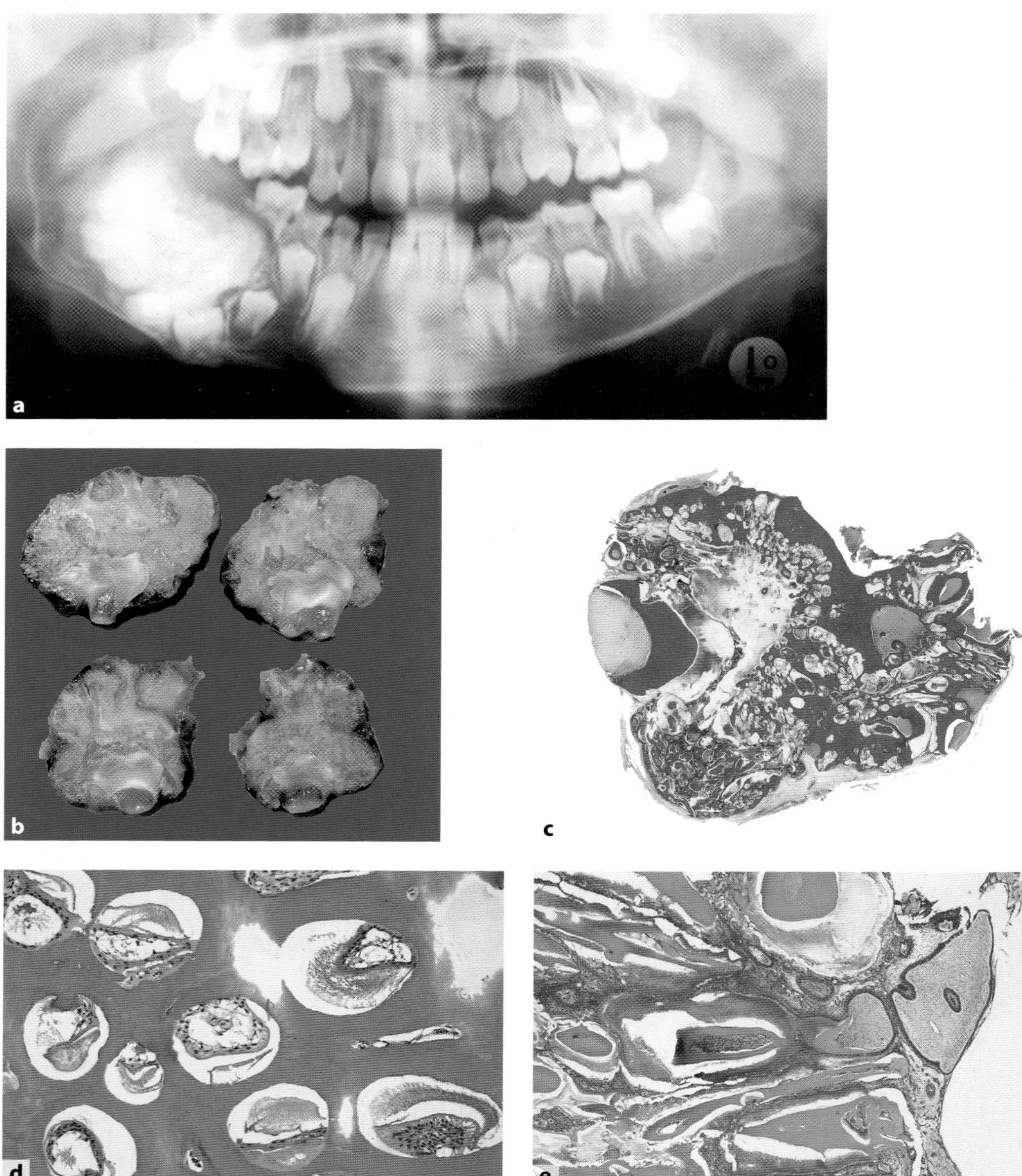

Fig. 10.17a–e Complex odontoma. **a** Radiograph showing calcified tissue mass coronally to a tooth germ. It is understandable that this condition will hamper normal tooth eruption. (From [13], with permission) **b** Cut surface showing gross appearance of tooth germ surrounded by hard tissue mass. **c** Low power view of same lesion as shown in **b**. The mixture of dental hard and soft tissue is arranged haphazardly without any resemblance to a tooth. **d** Micrograph showing dentin mass with cavities in which remnants of enamel matrix can be seen. **e** Detail from **c** to show the active formation of enamel and dentin. Odontogenic soft tissues are present but to a lesser extent than in ameloblastic fibro-odontoma

Odontoma-like structures may also occur in the hyperplastic dental follicle (see Chap. 11). Not yet completely matured complex odontomas may display the same mixture of soft and hard odontogenic tissues as shown by ameloblastic fibro-odontoma but usually, the hard tissues dominate the picture in the odontoma and play only a minor role in the ameloblastic fibro-odontoma. Sometimes, however, the distinction may remain a matter of personal preference due to overlapping features.

10.3.4 Odontoma—Compound Type

Compound odontoma is a malformation consisting of tiny teeth that may vary in number from only a few to numerous (Fig. 10.18). These teeth do not resemble normal teeth, but are usually cone-shaped. Histologically, they show the normal arrangement of centrally placed fibrovascular pulp tissue surrounded by dentin with an outer surface covered by enamel in the crown area and cementum in the root part.

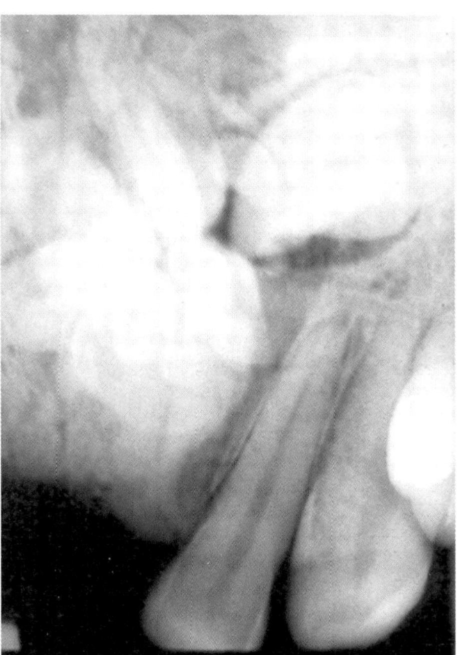

Fig. 10.18 Compound odontoma. Radiograph showing the admixture of structures recognisable as tiny teeth

10.3.5 Odonto-Ameloblastoma

Odonto-ameloblastoma is a very rare neoplasm that combines the features of ameloblastoma and odontoma, including the presence of enamel and dentin [2].

10.3.6 Calcifying Odontogenic Cyst

In its most simple form, calcifying odontogenic cyst is a cavity with a fibrous wall and an epithelial lining. This epithelial lining closely mimics that seen in unicystic ameloblastoma, but, in addition, there are intraepithelial eosinophilic ghost cells lacking nuclei that may undergo calcification. Ghost cell masses may also herniate through the basal lamina to reach the underlying stroma where they can act as foreign material and evoke a giant cell reaction (Figs. 10.19a, b). In the fibrous stroma adjacent to the basal epithelial cells, homogenous eosinophilic material resembling dentin may be found in varying amounts. Dentin-like material and ghost cells together may form mixed aggregates. To this simple unicystic structure other features may be added, thus creating different subtypes with different names.

The *proliferative calcifying odontogenic cyst* shows multiple intramural daughter cysts with an epithelial lining similar to the main cyst cavity. The *solid (neoplastic) calcifying odontogenic cyst* has been described by a variety of other terms: *dentinogenic ghost cell tumour, epithelial odontogenic ghost cell tumour, calcifying ghost cell odontogenic tumour,* and *cystic calcifying odontogenic tumour* [6, 16]. This lesion combines the morphology of an ameloblastoma with intraepithelial and stromal ghost cells with a dentin-like material. The most recent WHO classification proposes the diagnostic designations *calcifying cystic odontogenic tumour* and *dentinogenic ghost cell tumour* to discern between the cystic and the

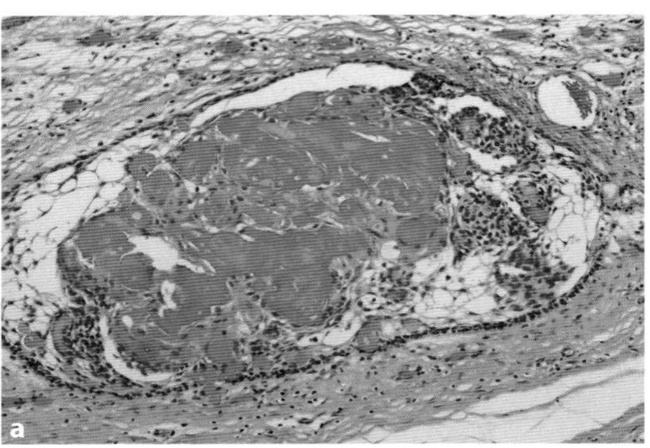

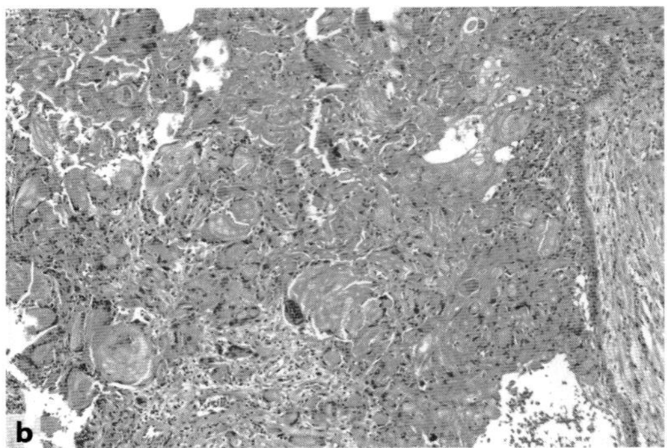

Fig. 10.19a,b Calcifying odontogenic cyst (Calcifying cystic odontogenic tumour) showing cyst lining similar to ameloblastoma but also containing ghost cells. Ghost cells may form a minor component (**a**) or extensive masses protruding into the stroma and evoking a giant cell reaction (**b**)

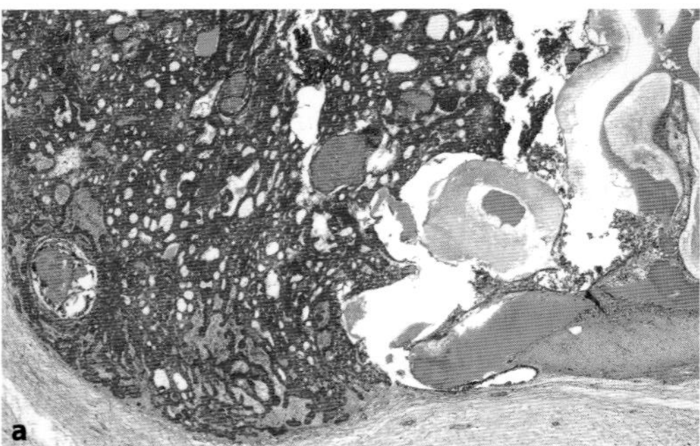

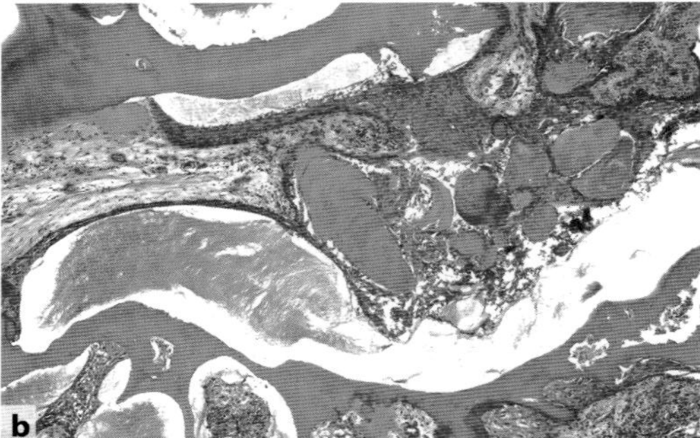

Fig. 10.20a,b Calcifying odontogenic cyst in combination with immature complex odontoma. Ameloblastic epithelium containing ghost cells (**a**) as well as immature odontogenic tissues with deposition of enamel and dentin (**b**) are present

solid lesion [2]. Also, calcifying odontogenic cysts may occur in association with other odontogenic tumours, in most instances ameloblastoma and odontoma (Figs. 10.20a, b) [16]. Ghost cells, either intraepithelially or in the stroma, allow the distinction between calcifying odontogenic cyst and ameloblastoma. The solid variant of calcifying odontogenic cyst is similar to craniopharyngioma [1].

10.4 Odontogenic Tumours—Malignant

Both odontogenic epithelium as well as odontogenic mesenchyme may show neoplastic degeneration, resulting in either odontogenic carcinomas or odontogenic sarcomas [11]. All entities to be mentioned show the clinical presentation and course as well as the radiographic appearance of an intraosseous malignant tumour.

10.4.1 Malignant Ameloblastoma

Malignant (metastasizing) ameloblastoma is an ameloblastoma that metastasizes in spite of an innocuous histologic appearance. The primary tumour shows no specific features that are different from ameloblastomas that do not metastasize. Therefore, this diagnosis can only be made in retrospect, after the occurrence of metastatic

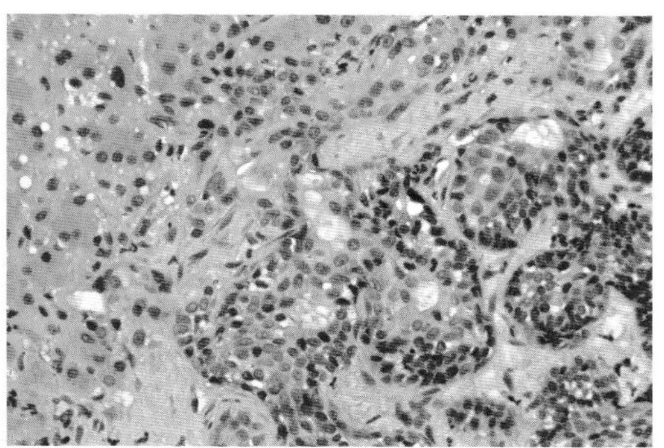

Fig. 10.21 Malignant ameloblastoma: metastasis of ameloblastoma in liver

deposits (Fig. 10.21). It is thus clinical behaviour and not histology that justifies a diagnosis of malignant ameloblastoma [11].

10.4.2 Ameloblastic Carcinoma

Ameloblastic carcinoma is characterised by cells that, although mimicking the architectural pattern of ameloblastoma, exhibit pronounced cytological atypia and mitotic activity, thus allowing the distinction between ameloblastic carcinoma and ameloblastoma (Fig. 10.22). Metastatic lesions are described in the lungs and in the lymph nodes.

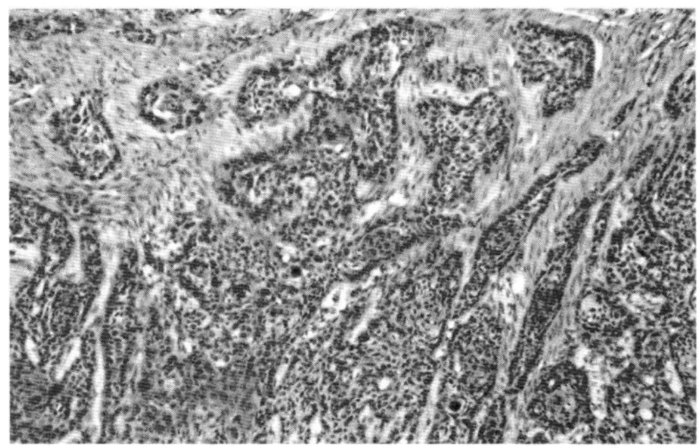

Fig. 10.22 Ameloblastic carcinoma combining islands with peripheral cylindrical cells as in ameloblastoma with cytonuclear atypia indicating malignancy

10.4.3 Primary Intraosseous Carcinoma

Primary intraosseous carcinoma is a squamous cell carcinoma arising within the jaw, having no initial connection with the oral mucosa, and presumably developing from residues of the odontogenic epithelium. The tumour may arise from a still recognisable precursor lesion such as the epithelial lining of an odontogenic cyst. Also, enamel epithelium has been documented as a tissue of origin [11].

10.4.4 Clear Cell Odontogenic Carcinoma

Clear cell odontogenic carcinoma is composed of cells with clear cytoplasm. These cells form nests and strands, intermingled with smaller islands of cells with eosinophilic cytoplasm (Figs. 10.23a–c).

10.4.5 Ghost Cell Odontogenic Carcinoma

Ghost odontogenic cell carcinoma, also called *malignant epithelial odontogenic ghost cell tumour* is a tumour that combines the elements of a benign calcifying odontogenic cyst with a malignant epithelial component (Figs. 10.24a, b). Only a few cases of this tumour have been reported, thus precluding any conclusions regarding clinicopathologic features. The tumour apparently arises most often from malignant transformation of a pre-existing benign calcifying odontogenic cyst.

10.4.6 Odontogenic Sarcoma

The WHO discerns between ameloblastic fibrosarcoma, ameloblastic fibrodentino- and fibro-odontosarcoma, and odontogenic carcinosarcoma [2]. The *ameloblastic fibrosarcoma* consists of malignant connective tissue admixed with epithelium similar to that seen in an ameloblastoma

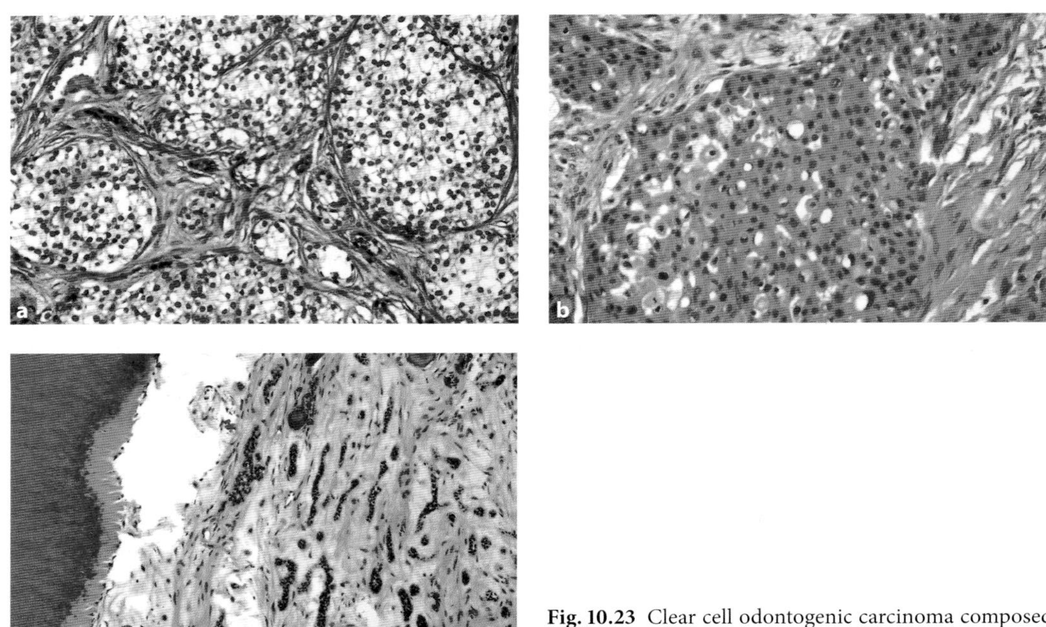

Fig. 10.23 Clear cell odontogenic carcinoma composed of clear cells (**a**) and eosinophilic cells (**b**). Tumour cells have invaded the pulp which is very rarely seen (**c**)

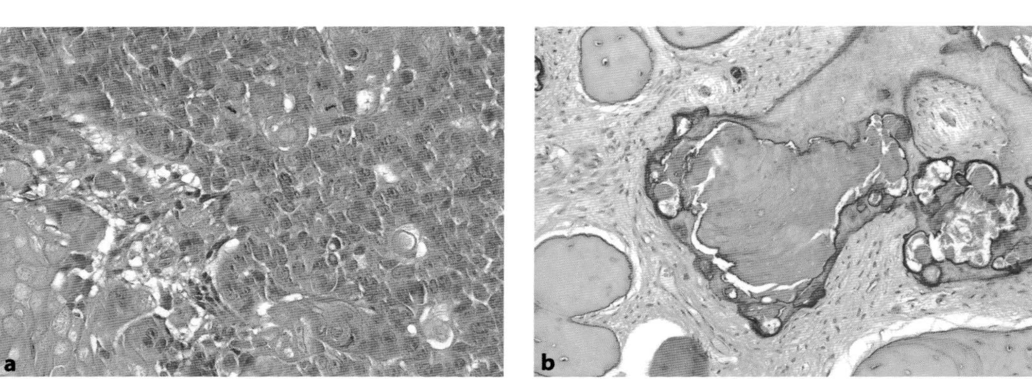

Fig. 10.24a,b Photomicrograph showing ghost cell odontogenic carcinoma. **a** Combination of soft tissue component resembling ameloblastic carcinoma but with also deposition of giant cells. **b** Stromal induction results in the formation of large cementum-like deposits

or ameloblastic fibroma. If there is also dentin, this is known as an *ameloblastic fibrodentinosarcoma*, and if there is also enamel, it is called *ameloblastic fibro-odontosarcoma*. This subclassification has no prognostic significance [11]. Those extremely rare lesions that combine carcinomatous and sarcomatous elements, but are recognisable as odontogenic through their epithelial component resembling ameloblastic carcinomas, have been called *odontogenic carcinosarcoma* or *odontogenic carcinoma with sarcomatous proliferation* [2, 11].

References

1. Badger JV, Gardner DG (1997) The relationship of adamantinomatous craniopharyngioma to ghost cell ameloblastoma of the jaws: a histopathologic and immunohistochemical study. J Oral Pathol Med 26:349–355
2. Barnes L, Eveson JW, Reichart PA et al. (eds) World Health Organization Classification of Tumours (2005) Pathology and genetics of tumours of the head and neck. Chapter 6. Odontogenic tumours. IARC, Lyon. pp 283–327
3. Calvo N, Alonso D, Prieto M et al. (2002) Central odontogenic fibroma granular cell variant: a case report and review of the literature. J Oral Maxillofac Surg 60:1192–1194
4. Gorlin RJ, Goltz RW (1960) Multiple nevoid basal cell epithelioma, jaw cysts and bifid rib. A syndrome. N Engl J Med 262:908–912
5. Kim J, Ellis GL (1993) Dental follicular tissue: misinterpretation as odontogenic tumors. J Oral Maxillofac Surg 51:762–767
6. Li TJ, Yu SF (2003) Clinicopathologic spectrum of the so-called calcifying odontogenic cysts. A study of 21 intraosseous cases with reconsideration of the terminology and classification. Am J Surg Pathol 27:372–384
7. Lukinmaa PL, Hietanen J, Anttinen J, et al. (1990) Contiguous enlarged dental follicles with histologic features resembling the WHO type of odontogenic fibroma. Oral Surg Oral Med Oral Pathol 70:313–317
8. Müller H, Slootweg PJ (1988) A peculiar finding in Le Fort I osteotomy. J Craniomaxillofac Surg 16:238–239
9. Philipsen HP, Reichart PA, Praetorius F (1997) Mixed odontogenic tumours and odontomas. Considerations on interrelationship. Review of the literature and presentation of 134 cases of odontomas. Oral Oncol 33:86–99
10. Sharpe PT (2001) Neural crest and tooth morphogenesis. Adv Dent Res 15:4–7
11. Slootweg PJ (2002) Malignant odontogenic tumors; an overview. Mund Kiefer Gesichtschir 6:295–302
12. Slootweg PJ (2006) MINI-SYMPOSIUM: HEAD AND NECK PATHOLOGY. Odontogenic tumours —An update. Current Diagnostic Pathology; 12:54–65
13. Slootweg PJ (2006) Chapter 4. Maxillofacial skeleton and teeth. In: Cardesa A, Slootweg PJ (eds) Pathology of the head and neck, Springer, Berlin-Heidelberg. p 115
14. Suarez PA, Batsakis JG, El-Naggar AJ (1996) Pathology consultation. Don't confuse dental soft tissues with odontogenic tumors. Ann Otol Rhinol Laryngol 105:490–494
15. Thesleff I, Keränen S, Jernvall J (2001) Enamel knots as signaling centers linking tooth morphogenesis and odontoblast differentiation. Adv Dent Res 15:14–18
16. Toida M (1998) So-called calcifying odontogenic cyst: review and discussion on the terminology and classification. J Oral Pathol Med 27:49–52

Chapter 11

Immature Odontogenic Tissues. A Source of Diagnostic Confusion

11

11.1 Introduction

As already mentioned, immature odontogenic tissues may closely mimic odontogenic tumours. Quite often, it may be very difficult to decide if the structures visible in the slide are indicating the presence of an odontogenic tumour or if they are just remnants of tissues connected with tooth development. Two different parts of the immature tooth are important in this respect: the dental papilla and the dental follicle. Both will be discussed in some detail.

First, it has to be emphasised that one should be very cautious in making a diagnosis of some kind of odontogenic tumour on tissue taken from a jaw area still containing developing teeth and not showing any clinical or radiographic sign of tumour being present. The ubiquitousness of immature odontogenic tissues in the jaw of children is shown in Fig. 11.1. This picture illustrates that the chance of encountering immature odontogenic tissues in tissue samples from this area and at this age is rather high.

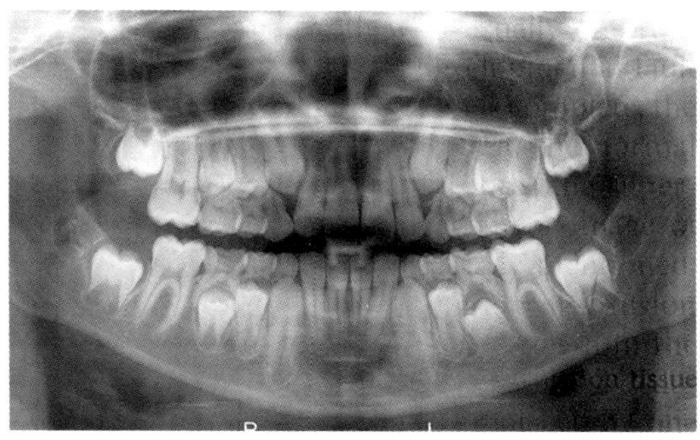

Fig. 11.1 Radiograph showing mixed dentition. Germs of the permanent teeth in varying stages of maturation are seen in upper and lower jaw. The 3rd molar germ just has started to form dental hard tissues whereas the 2nd permanent molar germ shows a very pronounced radiolucent rim representing the dental follicle. Other tooth germs show wide apical foramina indicating incompletely formed roots. Histologic details from this root area are shown in Fig. 11.2

11.2 Dental Papilla

The dental papilla is the mesenchymal soft tissue part of the tooth germ. During development and maturation, it gradually transforms into the dental pulp. Concomitant with this transformation, it decreases in volume and changes its histomorphology from mainly myxoid to more fibrous. Due to this myxoid nature, the dental papilla can be mistaken for odontogenic myxoma with serious consequences for the patient [5, 12].

This diagnostic pitfall can be avoided by an enquiry into the source of the tissue. If there is evidence that it comes from the vicinity of a developing tooth, dental papilla is much more likely to be the appropriate diagnosis than odontogenic myxoma. Moreover, in case of dental papilla, the myxoid tissue quite often is accompanied by some strands of odontogenic epithelium representing remnants of the enamel organ and also, it may show a peripheral cell condensation indicating presence of odontoblasts. Finally, a shell of dentin adjacent to the myxoid tissue may be helpful in differentiating odontogenic myxoma from dental papilla (Figs. 11.2, 11.3a–d).

In practice, this diagnostic pitfall especially applies to biopsies taken from elevations of the bottom of the maxillary sinus. These elevations may well represent the cranial part of developing maxillary tooth germs. If biopsied and submitted as tissue from a swelling in the maxillary sinus, an erroneous diagnosis of maxillary odontogenic myxoma is easily made [6].

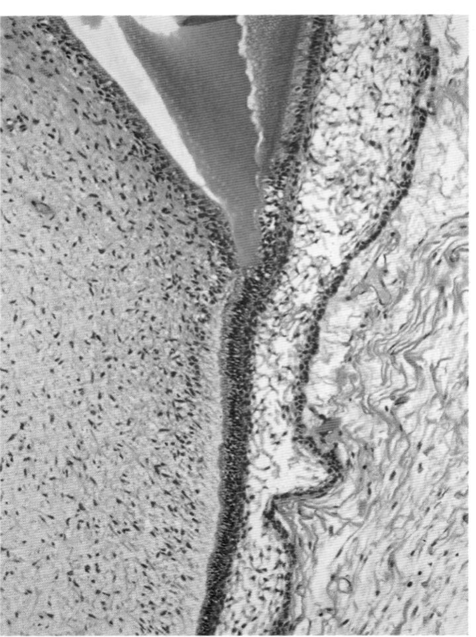

Fig. 11.2 Photomicrograph of the apical part of a tooth germ. Dental papilla (*left side*) consisting of immature myxoid connective tissue faces dentin and inner enamel epithelium (*right side*). Interposed cell condensation represents layer of odontoblasts forming dentin. See also figures in Chap. 1

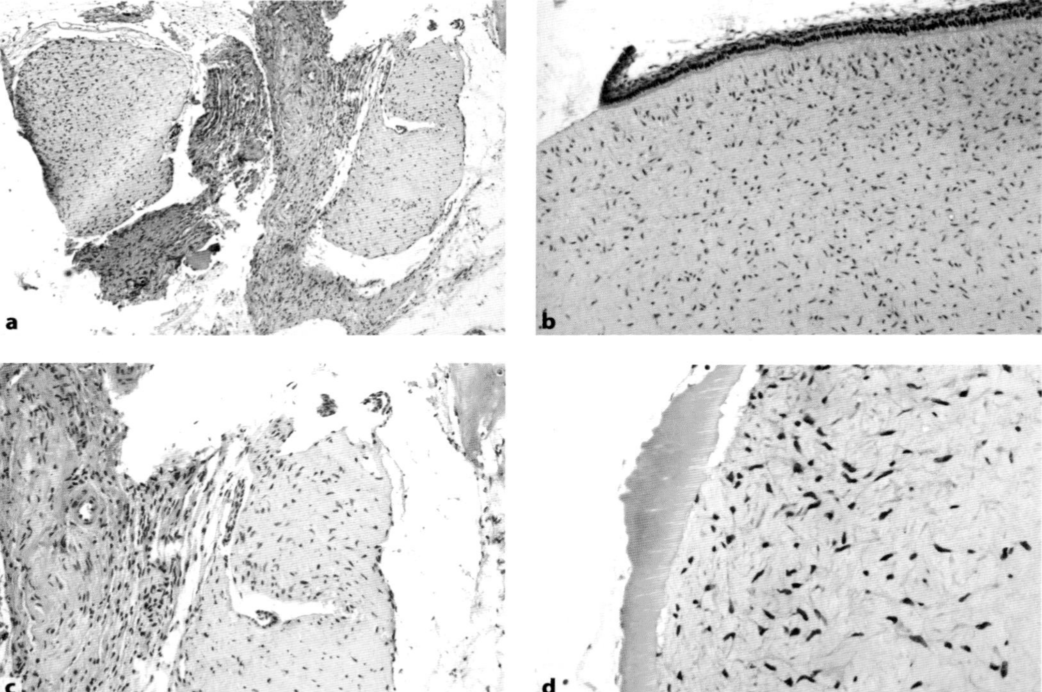

Fig. 11.3 Dental papilla mimicking myxoma. **a** Low power view showing fragments of loose myxoid tissue surrounded by more dense fibrous bands. **b** Adjacent strand of inner enamel epithelium reveals that it concerns a dental papilla and not a myxoma. **c** Sometimes, the epithelial component is only rudimentary. **d** Adjacent tubular dentin also indicates that it does not concern a myxoma but normal immature odontogenic tissue

11.3 Dental Follicle

The dental follicle is the fibrous sac that surrounds the not-yet-erupted immature tooth (Figs. 11.4a, b). At radiographs, it can be seen as a radiolucent rim surrounding the tooth germ (Fig. 11.1). Sometimes, this rim is larger than usually seen. This may lead to examination, including biopsy. As these dental follicles may consist of myxoid tissue, they may be mistaken for myxoma similar to that for the dental pulp [3, 12]. However, they may also contain a lot of other tissue components derived from the odontogenic apparatus including cementum, bone, dystrophic calcifications and nests, and strands of odontogenic epithelium. The arrangement of these tissues may simulate a variety of odontogenic tumours, either epithelial, mesenchymal, or mixed as illustrated in Figs. 11.5a–h. Again, it should be emphasised that these pictures encountered in tissues taken from the vicinity of a tooth germ should never

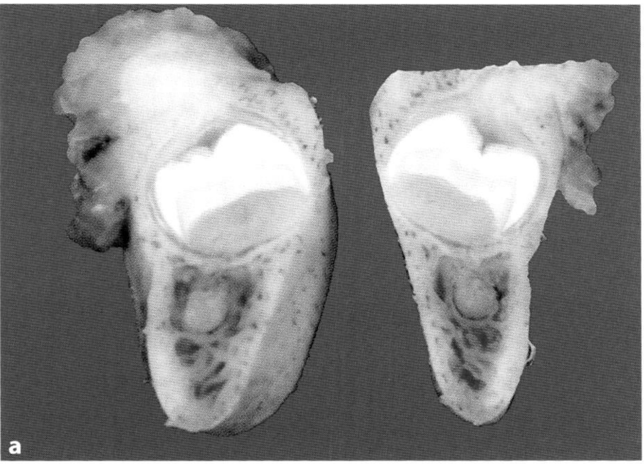

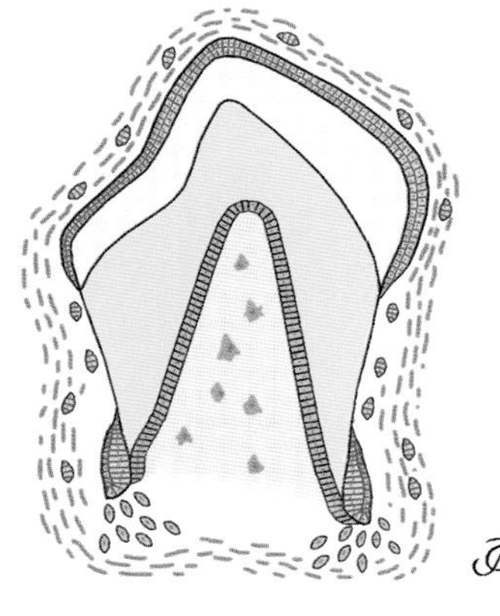

Fig. 11.4 **a** Cut surface showing tooth germ in its bony crypt. The fibrous capsule that surrounds this tooth germ represents the dental follicle. **b** Schematic drawing of tooth germ with surrounding follicle. (Drawing by John A.M. de Groot)

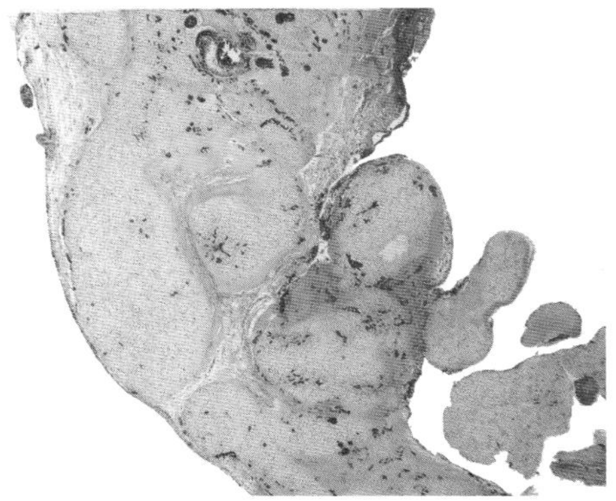

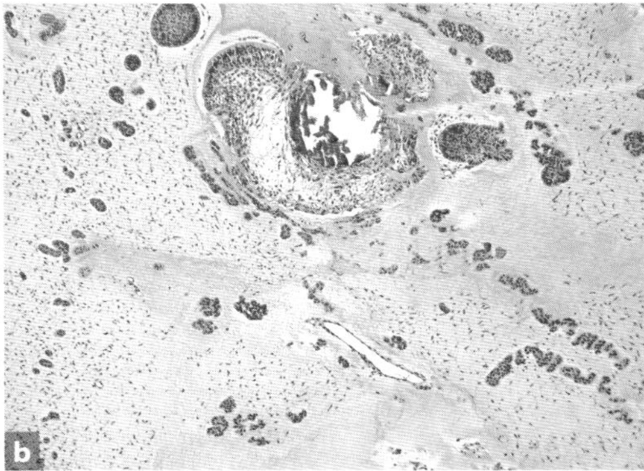

Fig. 11.5a–h Hyperplastic dental follicle may contain immature odontogenic tissues simulating odontogenic tumours. **a** Nodules of myxoid tissue with dispersed odontogenic epithelium mimicking ameloblastic fibroma. However, the nodular arrangement precludes that diagnosis as does the absence of any clinical sign of tumour. **b** Higher magnification showing formation of dental hard tissues adjacent to epithelium thus mimicking ameloblastic fibro-odontoma. **c** *see next page*

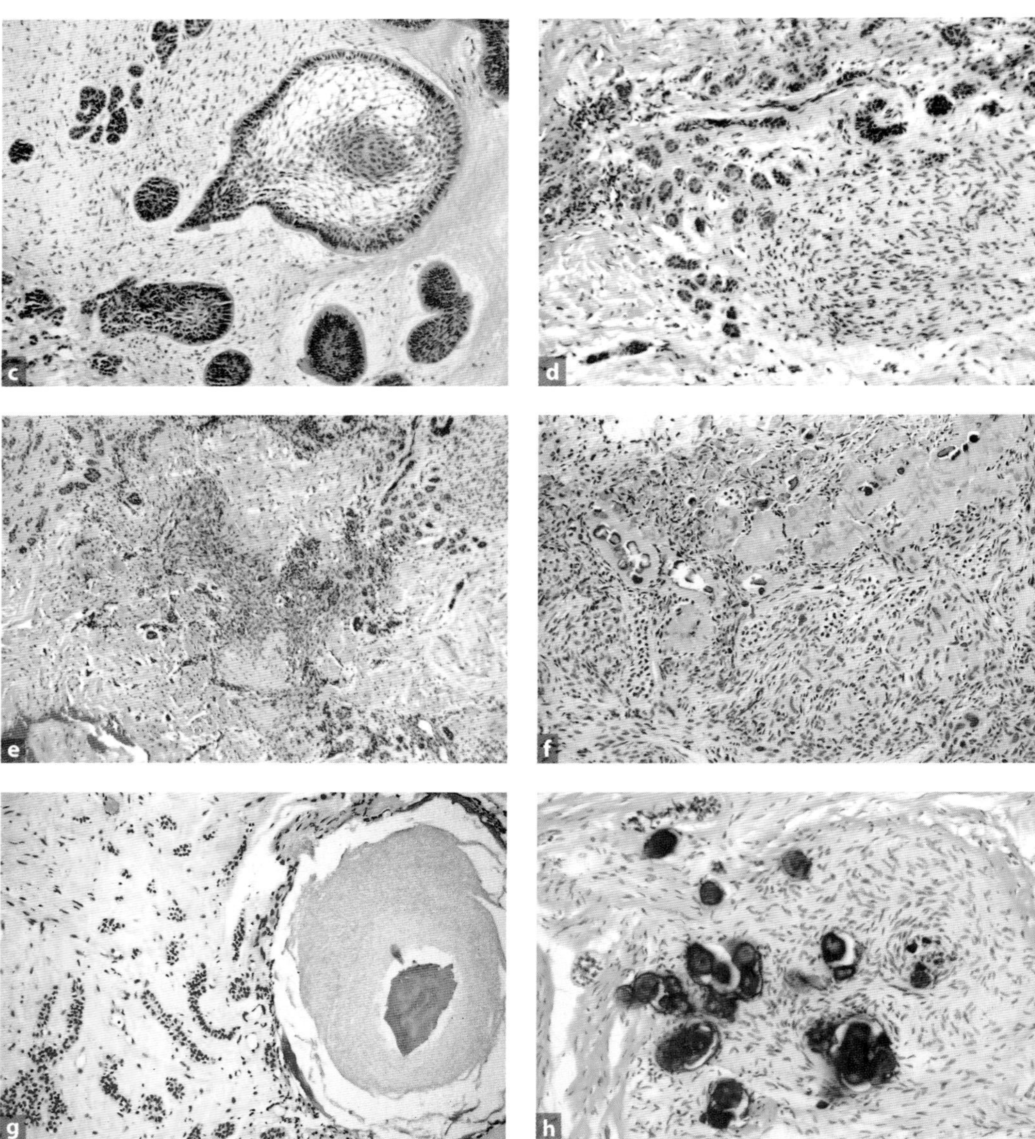

Fig. 11.5 *(continued)* Hyperplastic dental follicle may contain immature odontogenic tissues simulating odontogenic tumours. **c** Higher magnification showing epithelial nests resembling ameloblastoma. However, coexistence of immature myxoid tissue indicates either ameloblastic fibroma or a hamartomatous component of a dental follicle. **d** Cell-rich area of odontogenic mesenchyme with dispersed epithelial nests. **e** Mixture of more myxoid and more fibrous parts of the dental follicle together with many epithelial remnants. **f** Deposition of dysplastic dentin in cell-rich area of odontogenic mesenchyme. **g** Particle consisting of dentin core covered with immature enamel and surrounded by immature odontogenic epithelium and mesenchyme. **h** Dystrophic calcifications formed in association with odontogenic mesenchyme

been taken as evidence for neoplasia in the absence of clinical or radiologic signs suggesting tumour growth. They should be considered hamartomatous tissue alterations connected with tooth development.

Sometimes, enlarged dental follicles may be associated with multiple unerupted teeth [2, 4, 11]. Moreover, unerupted teeth with large pericoronal fibrous lesions may occur together with other dental abnormalities such as enamel dysplasia and pulpal calcifications [1, 8, 10].

Finally, odontogenic hamartomatous lesions may be found in the so-called opercula, the soft tissue barrier lying between the oral cavity and the crown of the erupting tooth. In case of delayed tooth eruption, the oral surgeon may excise this soft tissue mass that consists of both gingival fibrous tissue and the adjacent part of the underlying dental follicle for exposure of the tooth crown and thus facilitating subsequent eruption. Histologic examination of these opercula should be done with the same caveats as already mentioned [7, 9].

References

1. Feller L, Jadwat Y, Bouckaert M et al. (2006) Enamel dysplasia with odontogenic fibroma-like hamartomas. Review of the literature and report of a case. Oral Surg Oral Med Oral Pathol Oral Radiol Endod 101:620–624
2. Gardner DG, Radden B (1995) Multiple calcifying hyperplastic dental follicles. Oral Surg Oral Med Oral Pathol Oral Radiol Endod 79:603–606
3. Kim J, Ellis GL (1993) Dental follicular tissue: misinterpretation as odontogenic tumors. J Oral Maxillofac Surg 51:762–767
4. Lukinmaa PL, Hietanen J, Anttinen J et al. (1990) Contiguous enlarged dental follicles with histologic features resembling the WHO type of odontogenic fibroma. Oral Surg Oral Med Oral Pathol 70:313–317
5. Massey D (2005) Potential pitfalls in diagnostic oral pathology. A review for the general surgical pathologist. Adv Anat Pathol 12:332–349
6. Müller H, Slootweg PJ (1988) A peculiar finding in Le Fort I osteotomy. J Craniomaxillofac Surg 16:238–239
7. Onishi T, Sakashita S, Ogawa T et al. (2003) Histopathological characteristics of eruption mesenchymal calcified hamartoma: two case reports. J Oral Pathol Med 32:246–249
8. Peters E, Cohen M, Altini M (1992) Rough hypoplastic amelogenesis imperfecta with follicular hyperplasia. Oral Surg Oral Med Oral Pathol Oral Radiol Endod 74:87–92
9. Philipsen HP, Thosaporn W, Reichart PA et al. (1992) Odontogenic lesions in opercula of permanent molars delayed in eruption. J Oral Pathol Med 21:38–41
10. Raubenheimer EJ, Noffke CE (2002) Central odontogenic fibroma-like tumors, hypodontia, and enamel dysplasia: Review of the literature and report of a case. Oral Surg Oral Med Oral Pathol Oral Radiol Endod 94:74–77
11. Sandler HJ, Nersanian RR, Cataldo E et al. (1988) Multiple dental follicles with odontogenic fibroma-like changes (WHO type). Oral Surg Oral Med Oral Pathol 66:78–84
12. Suarez PA, Batsakis JG, El-Naggar AJ (1996) Pathology consultation. Don't confuse dental soft tissues with odontogenic tumors. Ann Otol Rhinol Laryngol 105:490–494

Subject Index

Printing: Krips bv, Meppel
Binding: Stürtz, Würzburg